# Praise for
## *Hospice & Palliative Care Handbook*, Third Edition

"While the core mission of hospice and palliative care remains to minimize suffering and optimize quality of life, the field has undergone sweeping changes in recent years. Today's hospice and palliative care practitioners are truly fortunate to be able to tap into Tina Marrelli's unparalleled clinical and operational expertise—as well as her rich historical perspectives on our nation's unique approach to end-of-life care. With the assistance of nationally recognized experts, Marrelli has expertly revised Hospice & Palliative Care Handbook, Third Edition. This book should be mandatory reading (and reference!) for hospice personnel."

–Theresa M. Forster
Vice President for Hospice Policy & Programs
National Association for Home Care & Hospice

"There has never been a more important time in hospice and palliative care for Tina Marrelli's invaluable manual. This book will guide both those new to this specialty field and those more veteran to meet the ever-increasing requirements for accurate, timely, and comprehensive documentation. The hospice and palliative care field is growing, and Marrelli's work provides an important resource to assist clinicians in meeting regulations while providing incredible care. This book is truly a must-have for all hospice and palliative caregivers."

–Soozi Flannigan, DNP, APRN
Vice President of Hospice & Home Care
The Connecticut Hospice Inc.

"I recommend this new edition as an excellent resource for professionals who are new to hospice and palliative care as well as a refresher for those who currently work in this specialty. Specific tips for success related to quality, safety, eligibility, and reimbursement are relevant to achieve quality patient care, comply with multiple federal and state regulations, and meet the educational needs of patients and caregivers."

–Marilyn D. Harris, MSN, RN, NEA-BC, FAAN
Former Executive Director of Hospice and Home Care
(Abington Hospital/Jefferson Health, Abington, Pennsylvania)
and Editor

D1070231

# HOSPICE & PALLIATIVE CARE HANDBOOK

## THIRD EDITION

Quality, Compliance, and Reimbursement

TINA M. MARRELLI

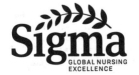

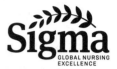

*The Honor Society of Nursing, Sigma Theta Tau International (STTI) is a nonprofit organization founded in 1922 whose mission is to support the learning, knowledge, and professional development of nurses committed to making a difference in health worldwide. Members include practicing nurses, instructors, researchers, policymakers, entrepreneurs, and others. STTI has more than 500 chapters located at more than 700 institutions of higher education throughout Armenia, Australia, Botswana, Brazil, Canada, Colombia, England, Ghana, Hong Kong, Japan, Kenya, Lebanon, Malawi, Mexico, the Netherlands, Pakistan, Portugal, Singapore, South Africa, South Korea, Swaziland, Sweden, Taiwan, Tanzania, Thailand, the United Kingdom, and the United States of America. More information about STTI can be found online at www.nursingsociety.org.*

**Sigma Theta Tau International**
**550 West North Street**
**Indianapolis, IN, USA 46202**

To order additional books, buy in bulk, or order for corporate use, contact Nursing Knowledge International at 888.NKI.4YOU (888.654.4968/US and Canada) or +1.317.634.8171 (outside US and Canada).

To request a review copy for course adoption, email solutions@nursingknowledge.org or call 888.NKI.4YOU (888.654.4968/US and Canada) or +1.317.634.8171 (outside US and Canada).

To request author information, or for speaker or other media requests, contact Marketing, Honor Society of Nursing, Sigma Theta Tau International at 888.634.7575 (US and Canada) or +1.317.634.8171 (outside US and Canada).

| **ISBN:** | 9781945157455 | **PDF ISBN:** | 9781945157479 |
| **EPUB ISBN:** | 9781945157462 | **MOBI ISBN:** | 9781945157486 |

---

Library of Congress Cataloging-in-Publication Data

Names: Marrelli, T. M., author. | Sigma Theta Tau International, issuing body.
Title: Hospice & palliative care handbook : quality, compliance, and reimbursement / Tina M. Marrelli.
Description: Third edition. | Indianapolis, IN, USA: Sigma Theta Tau International, [2018] | Includes bibliographical references and index.
Identifiers: LCCN 2017051743 (print) | LCCN 2017052072 (ebook) | ISBN 9781945157462 (Epub) | ISBN 9781945157479 (Pdf) | ISBN 9781945157486 (Mobi) | ISBN 9781945157455 (print : alk. paper) | ISBN 9781945157486 (mobi)
Subjects: | MESH: Hospice Care--standards | Palliative Care--standards | Documentation--standards | Quality Assurance, Health Care | Handbooks | Practice Guideline
Classification: LCC RA1000 (ebook) | LCC RA1000 (print) | NLM WB 39 | DDC 616.02/9--dc23
LC record available at https://lccn.loc.gov/2017051743

---

**First Printing, 2018**

| | |
| --- | --- |
| **Publisher:** Dustin Sullivan | **Principal Book Editor:** Carla Hall |
| **Acquisitions Editor:** Emily Hatch | **Development and Project Editor:** Rebecca Senninger |
| **Editorial Coordinator:** Paula Jeffers | **Copy Editor:** Gill Editorial Services |
| **Cover Designer:** Rebecca Batchelor | **Proofreader:** Todd Lothery |
| **Interior Design/Page Layout:** Bumpy Design | **Indexer:** Joy Dean Lee |

## ACKNOWLEDGMENTS

I would like to acknowledge and thank all the hospice nurses, therapists, pharmacists, physicians, aides, and many others whom I have known and worked with across decades. This is a thank-you to the many hospice (and home care) leaders and clinicians across many years who asked me great and interesting questions. As hospice has grown in its complexity, so too has the size of this third edition in pages!

A few people must be acknowledged.

Jennifer Kennedy for her contributions of time and lots of effort for this book to be updated, totally revised, and generally re-created. I have known Jennifer Kennedy, MA, BSN, RN, CHC, Senior Director, Regulatory and Quality, National Hospice and Palliative Care Organization (NHCPO) for more than 10 years. At that time, I had a hospice-specific question and met Jennifer. We have remained friends and colleagues ever since. Thank you so much, Jennifer!

I would also like to acknowledge Cat Armato, RN, CHPN, CHC, CHPC, Health Care Consultant, Armato & Associates, LLC for her kind sense of humor, formatting skills, clarity in writing, enhancement of content, meeting of deadlines, and more. Thank you, Cat!

Reviewers of a manuscript always strengthen and enhance the substance of a book, so I also thank the reviewers listed in the following "Reviewer" pages. Some of you have reviewed other editions, which speaks to the relationships forged in homecare and hospice organizations. "New eyes" are always a good thing, as there comes a time when one cannot "see" what was written.

I am heartened that, in hospice, we know and retain the fundamentals of the best care. This book is also dedicated to you—those mentoring, leading, and otherwise managing in hospice wherever it is provided—inspiring, mentoring, and otherwise helping clinicians be able to provide the best care for hospice patients and families.

# ABOUT THE AUTHOR

## Tina M. Marrelli, MSN, MA, RN, FAAN

Tina Marrelli is the author of numerous books, including *Home Care Nursing: Surviving in an Ever-Changing Care Environment*, her book directed toward caregivers, a sometimes undervalued person on the healthcare team; *A Guide for Caregiving: What's Next? Planning for Safety, Quality, and Compassionate Care for Your Loved One and Yourself!*; *Handbook of Home Health Standards: Quality, Documentation and Reimbursement* (2018); and *The Nurse Manager's Survival Guide*.

Tina has a long-term relationship with hospice and hospice colleagues. Medicare did not recognize hospices or pay for hospice care until 1982. In the early years of hospice, both the staff at CMS and the leaders of the early hospices worked to make sense of the law and the population it served, working together to develop the kind of hospice care that is now identified with the name. She was an early participant and remembers those heady days. For the more "experienced" readers, you might recall Tom Hoyer of HCFA (now CMS) fame. Tom was termed the "hospice czar" and was a driving force for positive change. This means that at that time, hospice was primarily volunteer. It was pretty much grassroots and mission-driven to try to change and improve end-of-life care for patients and to support their loved ones. This all sounds common sense now, but looking back, it was not. At that time, Tina was the Director of a systems-based nonprofit Home Care and Hospice in Annapolis, Maryland (USA), and it was the first hospice to receive TJC accreditation. So she has always embraced the hospice philosophy and model and (still) wonders why the rest of the healthcare system does not also embrace family and friend caregivers.

Tina attended Duke University School of Nursing, where she received her undergraduate degree in nursing. She also has a master's degree in health administration and in nursing. Tina has worked in hospitals, nursing homes, and public health. She has practiced as a visiting nurse and managed in-home care and hospice for many years.

Tina is the Chief Clinical Officer for Innovative Caregiving Solutions, LLC, an innovative e-caregiving technology (www.e-caregiving.com). Finally, caregiving and caregivers (loved ones, friends, partners, and others) are being recognized for their important contributions, knowledge, and roles. Tina can be contacted at info@e-caregiving.com.

Tina is an international healthcare consultant, specializing in home care, hospice, and community-based models of care. Tina and her team of specialized consultants have been practicing in the home care and hospice environments for more than 20 years.

Tina is a founding member of the International Home Care Nurses Organization (www.IHCNO.org), which was developed "to support a vibrant worldwide network of nurses to promote excellence in providing optimal care to patients living at home wherever they live in the world." The IHCNO was started with a small but "mighty" group of nursing leaders.

Tina has been the editor of three peer-reviewed publications—most recently for *Home Healthcare Nurse* (now *Home Healthcare Now*), and she is an Editor Emeritus. Tina also serves on the editorial boards of the *Journal of Community Health Nursing* and *The American Nurse*.

Tina has been married to her "Hubby," Bill, for 25 years and hopes for another 25!

Tina is a cat person, but their last one, Limpy Buttercup, went to kitty heaven. Stay tuned for the next kitty! Tina and Bill have walked the beaches on Sea Turtle Patrol for more than 20 years on the west coast of Florida. There is almost nothing as exciting as seeing these vestiges of the dinosaur era come ashore to lay their eggs and then see and watch their hatchlings, all species of which are either threatened or endangered.

# REVIEWERS

**Cathleen "Cat" Armato, RN, CHPN, CHC, CHPC**
Principal Consultant
Armato & Associates, LLC
Blairsville, Georgia

**Thomas Bradford, MSW**
Social Worker
Christiana Care
Visiting Nurse Association
New Castle, Delaware

**Dedee Cully, RN, LNC, COS-S**
CaseLNC Consulting
Republic, Missouri

**Warren Hebert, DNP, RN, CAE**
RWJF Executive Fellow
Chief Executive Officer
Homecare Association of Louisiana
Baton Rouge, Louisiana

**Jennifer Kennedy, MA, BSN, RN, CHC**
Senior Director, Regulatory and Quality
National Hospice and Palliative Care Organization
Alexandria, Virginia

**Daniel Maison, MD, FAAHPM, HMDC**
Lead Physician
Aspire Health
Grand Rapids, Michigan

# TABLE OF CONTENTS

# Foreword

I started my hospice career when pagers and a pocketful of quarters were "high-tech" communications. We knew where there were safe pay phones and a good place to get a cold bottle of Pepsi. Back in 1986, hospice had just become a permanent benefit under Medicare, and the foundation for the (then) Hospice Nurses Association (now known as the Hospice and Palliative Nurses Association) had not yet been laid.

I sometimes felt I was flying by the seat of my pants, and solid, comprehensive resource manuals weren't readily available. I often didn't know what I didn't know, but I had wonderful mentors and leaders to guide me as my career took root.

Fast forward 31 years, and I serve as a mentor to several professionals. One friend is ready to launch forward to that next step in leadership and is acutely aware of her knowledge gaps. Full of passion and a drive to succeed, she too is faced with sometimes not knowing what she doesn't know.

That's why I am glad to see that Tina Marrelli has once again updated her work in the third edition of *Hospice & Palliative Care Handbook*. Everyone who has been in hospice since 2013 has certainly felt the pain sometimes associated with the fast-paced regulatory changes. Perhaps it is fitting that this book was updated in 2017, which was a relatively quiet year for regulatory changes—a catch-up year for all of us!

So once again, a new generation of hospice professionals is learning the trade. New nurses are making sure they can document eligibility. New social workers or chaplains are reminded that their work (and the supporting documentation) is just as important—or sometimes more important—to the family. New hospice leaders who have worked in only one part of an organization are now ready to take the big leap to the chief executive role. All hospice professionals share the need to have an accurate understanding of hospice care at their fingertips.

To those colleagues of mine: Keep this manual handy as you create the future of hospice. It is your turn to care for us.

Thanks, Tina, for doing it again!

*–Kenneth Zeri, RN, MS*
*President & Chief Professional Officer, Hospice Hawaii*
*Past President, Hospice and Palliative Nurses Association (HPNA)*
*Board of Directors, National Hospice and*
*Palliative Care Association (NHPCO)*

# Preface

This book is in its third edition. The second, last edition, was published in 2005. So much has happened to hospice from regulatory, growth, and other perspectives. This newest edition is dedicated to all the clinicians and managers who make hospice the special way of caring for people and their families that it is. Hospice operations demand a commitment and attention to detail rarely found in other businesses or work settings.

This book is for the nurses, physicians, aides, pharmacists, chaplains, and others providing spiritual care, and other team members who provide important care while meeting often difficult and multilevel regulations.

This also acknowledges everyone in the office who support daily operations: the schedulers, on-call teams, administrative staff, quality improvement team members, human resource team members, educators, billers, sales people, CEOs, COOs, CFOs, executive directors, business/ corporate strategists, and customer service representatives—those who strive for "business as usual" whether there is an ice storm, a hurricane pending, a power outage, or any of numerous other events that affect patients and families and home care and hospice operations.

Thanks to all of you for what you contribute to the hospice profession every day!

The author can be contacted directly at info@e-caregiving.com.

# Introduction

The goal of this book is to help hospice clinicians, team members, and managers meet quality, coverage, and reimbursement standards and requirements in daily practice and operations and in documentation activities. The Hospice Care Guidelines or problem-specific topics are organized alphabetically for easy identification and retrieval of needed information. This information can then be individualized for your hospice patient/family and used throughout the clinical record. It can even serve as a basis for a common glossary in interdisciplinary (IDG) discussions and meetings. It is formatted and designed for easy review for care and care planning–related activities. The following information refers to the specifically numbered entries in each of the eight Hospice Care Guidelines.

*1. General Considerations.* This area contains general information about the health system problem and designated topic in relation to hospice care. There may also be symptoms listed as the basis for hospice care and care planning.

*2. Eligibility Considerations.* This section provides information to help support medical necessity from a quality and payer perspective. Hospice team members should stay apprised of changing regulatory information and should look to their specific Medicare Administrative Contractors (MACs) and their supervisors for more information.

*3. Potential Diagnoses ICD-10-CM Diagnostic Coding.* The International Statistical Classification of Diseases and Related Health Problems 10th Revision (ICD-10-CM) is a coding of diseases and signs, symptoms, abnormal findings, complaints, social circumstances, and external causes of injury or diseases, as classified by the World Health Organization (WHO). There are specific coding rules and conventions in the official coding manual that must be followed, and these rules may not be included in online websites or EMR software. Consult with a credentialed coder for any questions related to accurate coding. In this section, there are code ranges listed for that specific body system.

4. *Safety Considerations.* This section lists the general kinds of safety concerns that may impact hospice care, based on diagnoses, or the care guidelines listed. The information listed in safety considerations is to be used upon assessment and throughout the care and care planning–related processes.

5. *Skills and Services Identified.* This section lists and identifies the hospice team members and some of their specialized functions and interventions based on the patient's/family's diagnoses or problems and their unique circumstances. This section assists with the individualization of care, care planning, and documentation. These services include registered nurse, hospice aide, social worker, volunteer(s), spiritual counselor, and other services. This information is provided as a list to assist in the identification of needed hospice care and services and assists team members by identifying possible interventions and care based on the team member's education and professional scope of practice.

6. *Patient, Family, and Caregiver Educational Needs.* This section identifies care regimens that contribute to safe and effective care at home between the hospice team member's visits. This is a list of possible educational needs. This information is not all-inclusive and must be based on the patient's and family's unique circumstances and needs.

7. *Specific Tips for Quality, Safety, Eligibility, and Reimbursement.* These tips contribute to clear, specific documentation of care and care planning–related processes. These are oftentimes practical tips related to supporting medical necessity and individualizing documentation of hospice care.

*8. Quality Metrics.* The questions listed in this section were created to help clinicians and managers identify possible areas for coverage and improvement of care and related processes. Some of the questions help support medical necessity, while others are specific to assessment and other components of care. These questions could be incorporated into educational sessions or in other venues or opportunities to improve care, operations, and practice.

# Hospice Care: An Overview of Quality and Compassionate Care

Hospice, a type of palliative care, is considered to be the model for quality, compassionate care for people facing a life-limiting illness or injury. Hospice and palliative care involves an interdisciplinary team-oriented approach to expert medical and nursing care, pain and other symptom management, and emotional and spiritual support expressly tailored to the patient's unique needs and wishes (National Hospice and Palliative Care Organization [NHPCO], 2015a). Another special difference is that support is provided to the patient's loved ones as well. At the center of hospice and palliative care is the belief that each person has the right to die with dignity and in comfort. Families receive the necessary support to allow that to happen (NHPCO, 2015a). The patient, family, friends, and designee are the unit of care, not solely the patient. This is a very different and special construct seen primarily in hospice and palliative care.

The Centers for Medicare and Medicaid Services (CMS), the largest payer for hospice, defines hospice care as, "a comprehensive set of services identified and coordinated by an interdisciplinary group (IDG) to provide for the physical, psychosocial, spiritual, and emotional needs of a terminally ill patient and/or family members, as delineated in a specific patient plan of care" (CMS, 2008, p. 18).

The hospice philosophy of care asserts the concept of palliative care, which promotes quality of life by enhancing comfort for individuals and their families, whom hospice considers the unit of care. Hospice focuses on care versus cure. When a cure is no longer an option, hospice recognizes and provides support for a comfortable death with dignity as a fundamental goal of care. The hospice philosophy also recognizes that death is a part of the life cycle, and the provision of comprehensive palliative care that addresses pain relief and comfort enhances quality of life for the terminally ill. Hospice also acknowledges the possibility for growth of the individual and his/her family, and during the dying experience, the hospice team works to protect and nurture this potential (NHPCO, 2013b). The hospice team assesses the needs of the individual and the individual's family in the last phase of life and works with them collectively to develop a care approach that encompasses the physical, emotional, spiritual, and cultural concerns and wishes of the individual and the individual's family. Hospice provides palliative care to all individuals regardless of age, gender, cultural background, beliefs, diagnosis, availability of a caregiver, or ability to pay. Care is generally provided in the late stages of an advanced illness, during the dying process, and in the bereavement period.

Hospice core values include:

- Patient- and family-centered care
- Holistic relief of suffering
- Interdisciplinary team approach
- Ethical behavior
- Service excellence (NHPCO, 2013a)

## HISTORY OF HOSPICE

The word *hospice* can be traced back to the medieval era when it referred to a place of rest or shelter for tired or ill travelers who were on a long journey. Dame Cicely Saunders applied this term to her work with terminally ill patients in 1948 with her specialized approach to caring for the dying. Saunders developed the total pain theory to address the entirety of suffering (physical, spiritual, psychological, and social) for patients with advanced illness and at the end of life. Addressing a patient's pain in this holistic manner led to the provision of palliative care for patients with life-limiting illness. She also founded St. Christopher's Hospice, the first contemporary hospice, in London, and she is the matriarch of the modern hospice movement in the United States (Goebel et al., 2009). Saunders traveled to the Yale University School of Nursing in 1963 by invitation of Florence Wald, the Dean of Nursing, to introduce this unique type of care provision. In her series of lectures to medical students, nurses, social workers, and chaplains, she discussed the provision of holistic hospice care and included before and after photographs of patients with cancer to illustrate the impact of effective palliative symptom management. Dame Saunders's visit ultimately led to the start of the hospice movement in the United States and the formation of the first hospice in Connecticut, USA, which began serving patients in 1973 (Connor, 2008).

## HOSPICE AND HOSPICE GROWTH

There were hospices providing mission-driven skillful hospice care for patients and families years before Medicare and other reimbursement. Hospice has grown substantially in the United States. When hospice began in the States in the 1970s, cancer was the primary diagnosis for patients who accessed this unique type of care at the end of life. Medicare started reimbursing hospice care in 1983. In its growth and expansion throughout the decades, patients experiencing end stages of chronic diseases are now accessing hospice care, as are patients with cancer.

Some of the common end stage noncancer diagnoses include:

- ALS and other neurologic conditions
- Dementia due to Alzheimer's disease and related disorders
- Heart disease
- HIV disease
- Liver disease
- Pulmonary disease

- Renal disease
- Stroke
- Coma

In the March 2016 report to Congress, MedPAC (the Medicare Payment Advisory Commission, a nonpartisan legislative branch agency that provides the U.S. Congress with analysis and policy advice on the Medicare program) stated that hospice utilization increased across nearly all demographic populations. However, use remained low for racial and ethnic minority groups as compared to Caucasians (MedPAC, 2015). Hospice growth in terms of access and presence in the healthcare system over the past decade has primarily been attributed to:

- Reimbursement mechanisms by Medicare, Medicaid, and other payers
- The changing healthcare delivery system and fragmentation of services
- The growing number of frail and older adult individuals
- The shift from inpatient to outpatient and community-based care
- The change in hospice case mixes to include noncancer diagnoses
- The search for alternative care methods for advanced illnesses
- Increased engagement of patients by physicians related to advance care planning
- Changing belief systems of patients and their families relating to illness and death
- New communication technologies
- Growing recognition and support for family caregivers
- Development of quality measures to increase accountability
- Cost savings in the healthcare continuum

Medicare is the primary healthcare payer for hospice in the United States, and spending for hospice between 2000 and 2012 showed an over 400% increase. This was thought to be primarily driven by larger numbers of beneficiaries opting to use their hospice benefit and an increase in patient length of stay (MedPAC, 2015). Based on this substantial growth in hospice spending, the Affordable Care Act of 2010 included a provision for hospice payment reform, which was implemented in 2016. This is the first major change in how hospice care is reimbursed by Medicare since its inception in 1983.

## HOSPICE IN THE CARE CONTINUUM: WHERE DOES IT FIT?

As America's baby boomers age, comprehensive care in many different settings, including palliative care and end-of-life care, is needed. Hospice, as a type of palliative care, is part of the healthcare continuum. Hospice may be a stand-alone organization or part of a larger healthcare system, and it may be for-profit or not-for-profit.

In the past 100 years, life expectancy in the United States increased from 47 to 78 years, and there is a growing trend of individuals over the age of 90 years (Institute of Medicine, 2014). In a seamless care continuum, all healthcare providers work together to develop a coordinated patient plan of care that encompasses physical, emotional, social, spiritual, caregiving, nutritional, safety, and other needs. Hospice professionals are experts in providing care for individuals with a serious life-limiting illness. They have the capacity to assess the need for supportive services in their communities with the goal of developing and integrating into a unified continuum of care (NHPCO, 2013).

## WHAT IS A TERMINAL ILLNESS FROM A HOSPICE PERSPECTIVE?

An individual must be diagnosed with a terminal illness by a physician to qualify for hospice services. The Centers for Medicare and Medicaid Services (1983) defines the terminally ill as an individual who has a medical prognosis with a life expectancy of 6 months or less if the illness runs its normal course. Without focus on care issues such as pain and symptom management, an individual may experience increased suffering and isolation from loved ones. The provision of care that focuses on comfort and personal growth at the end of life is an option for individuals and their family through hospice care (NHPCO, 2013a).

## WHERE IS HOSPICE CARE PROVIDED?

Hospice care is provided to a patient and the patient's family wherever the patient calls home. These locations of care can include:

- Private home/residences
- Hospice residences
- Inpatient hospice facilities
- Nursing facilities (skilled nursing facility and long-term care facilities)
- Assisted living facilities
- Board and care homes (group homes)
- Hospitals (for acute symptom management)

Hospice is also distinctive because care provision does not need to take place in traditional healthcare settings. Studies show that roughly 80% of Americans prefer to die at home if possible. Despite this wish, 60% of Americans still die in hospitals, 20% die in nursing homes, and only 20% die at home (Stanford School of Medicine, 2016). There is clearly a disconnect between what patients want and where they receive care at the end of their lives.

The original intent of the 1983 Medicare Hospice Benefit (MHB) was to offer specialized physician services, nursing services, and other forms of supportive care in the home to enable a terminally ill individual to remain at home in the presence of family and friends as long as possible (CMS, 1983).

## THE HOSPICE INTERDISCIPLINARY GROUP: WHO ARE THEY?

Because hospice care is patient- and family-centered, the approach and care are accomplished with an interdisciplinary group (IDG) that, at a minimum, includes the hospice physician, nurse, social worker, counselors (bereavement, dietary), and spiritual care professional. These services are considered "core" services and must be provided to all patients and families. Additional noncore hospice team members include hospice aides; pharmacists; speech, physical, and occupational therapists (as needed); homemakers; and volunteers. All team members work together, with the patient's primary physician, focusing on the dying person's needs, whether those are physical, emotional, or spiritual (CMS, 2008). The goal of hospice care is to help keep the patient as pain- and symptom-free as possible, with loved ones nearby, and with the best quality of life possible. Most other settings in healthcare have a multidisciplinary approach, but the hospice interdisciplinary model of care delivery is mandated by law and embraced by the hospice team. Throughout this text, the term *interdisciplinary group* or *IDG* will be used, although *interdisciplinary team* or *IDT* is sometimes used in the industry.

## INTERDISCIPLINARY ROLES

The Medicare hospice Conditions of Participation (CoPs) are a framework required of Part A hospice providers and describe specific tenets of the hospice care and administration. These CoPs are discussed later in this chapter in more detail. One of the most important areas relates to the interdisciplinary group and its team members.

Each team member has a specific focus but works with other team members toward the common goals of hospice care.

- **Attending or primary physician**—The patient may or may not have an attending or primary physician. Having one is not a regulatory requirement. A patient has the right to choose their attending physician, and this right is a regulatory requirement in the Medicare hospice Conditions of Participation. The attending physician has an important role in the commencement and provision of hospice care and is considered a member of the hospice interdisciplinary group. The attending physician and the hospice medical director/hospice physician work closely together to determine and provide the best medical care for the patient through assessment of patient needs and administration of the patient's plan of care (NHPCO, 2011). The Medicare Hospice Benefit requires the attending physician to provide certification of a patient's terminal illness for the first 90-day benefit period (CMS, 2005).

**NOTE** State hospice licensure regulations for certification of terminal illness may be stricter. If that is the case, the hospice is obliged to adhere to the more stringent regulation. For questions or clarifications, check with your state hospice organization and state health department entity that manages survey and certification processes.

- **Nurse practitioners as attending physicians**—A nurse practitioner may serve as a patient's attending physician in hospice when the patient chooses the nurse practitioner as their attending physician. However, a nurse practitioner may not certify or recertify a patient's terminal illness. A nurse practitioner is defined as a registered nurse who is permitted to perform additional services as legally authorized in the state in which the nurse practitioner practices. Physician assistants are not recognized by the CMS to provide services within the Medicare Hospice Benefit (NHPCO, 2011).

## HOSPICE "CORE" SERVICES

The Medicare Hospice Benefit designates specific services as "core," which means that these services must be provided by a hospice employee and may not be routinely contracted. There are both core and noncore services. The noncore services are addressed in the next section.

Core services may only be contracted in temporary extraordinary circumstances, which could include unanticipated periods of increased patient census, staffing shortages due to illness or other short-term temporary circumstances that interrupt patient care, and temporary travel of a patient outside of the hospice's service area (CMS, 2008).

- **Hospice medical director and hospice physician**—While a hospice may employ one or more physicians through a direct employee, a contractual, or a volunteer relationship, there may be only one hospice medical director. Additional physicians function under the supervision of the hospice medical director. The single physician who serves in the role of the medical director assumes overall responsibility for the medical component of the hospice's patient care program. This responsibility includes supervision of the activity of physicians, nurses, social workers, therapists, and counselors within the hospice to ensure that these areas consistently meet patient and family needs.

The hospice program must also specify a physician designee who serves in the role of the medical director in his/her absence. All hospice physicians, in collaboration with the patient's attending physician, are responsible for the palliation and management of the diagnoses and conditions that contribute to the terminal prognosis. If the patient's attending physician is at any time unavailable, the medical director/hospice physician is responsible for meeting the medical needs of the patient (CMS, 2008). The medical director/ hospice physician serves as the physician member of the hospice IDG and provides initial certification and recertification of the terminal illness for hospice patients in collaboration with the patient's attending physician. This person serves as a resource for the attending physician and is available to assume the care of the patient per the patient's or attending physician's choice (NHPCO, 2011).

- **Nurse**—The clinical component of a patient's care is provided by and under the supervision of a registered nurse. The nurse assesses patient and family needs, implements medical orders from physicians, and serves as the manager of the patient's plan of care (CMS, 2008). Nurses provide clinical services that promote the palliative management of symptoms related to the terminal diagnosis and other related diagnoses and overall patient terminal prognosis. Interventions by the nurse include comprehensive assessment, medication administration and management, education of the patient and family about interventions and what to expect, and serving as the point of contact for the patient and family and the attending physician.

An effective hospice nurse should be skilled in physical assessment and management of pain and symptoms at the end of life. Hospice nurse educational backgrounds range from a 2-year nursing degree program to a master's degree.

Certification as a hospice and palliative care nurse is available through the Hospice & Palliative Credentialing Center in partnership with the Hospice & Palliative Nurses Association (HPNA). Certification is available to RNs, advanced-practice RNs (APRN), and licensed practical nurses/licensed vocational nurses (LPN/LVN) (Hospice & Palliative Credentialing Center, 2014). These certifications demonstrate the nurse's commitment to excellent and evidence-based practice.

If state regulations allow an RN, nurse practitioner, advanced-practice nurse, and others to see, treat, and write orders, then the RN may include these functions while providing nursing services for hospice patients. A hospice organization may use advance care nurses to enhance the nursing care furnished to its patients. An example of this type of advanced care nursing could include providing wound care and offering pediatric nurse specialists. Services offered by a nurse practitioner (NP) who is not the patient's attending physician are also included under nursing care. In addition, nurses are permitted to provide dietary counseling by federal regulation, but should the dietary needs of the patient exceed the expertise of the nurse, a dietary counselor must supply specialized care (CMS, 2008).

- **Social worker (SW)**—Social workers are an important component of the IDG. They provide emotional support, counseling, and resource identification. Services that social workers offer in hospice include financial assessment and planning, housing (placement in a facility), family and caregiver concerns, and funeral planning. A social worker may have a bachelor's or master's in social work, but the federal hospice regulations allow an individual with a baccalaureate degree in psychology, sociology, or another field related to social work to serve in the social work role. Baccalaureate degree social workers and individuals with a bachelor's in a related field must be supervised by a social worker with a master's degree (MSW).

> **NOTE** Social workers who have been employed with *the same hospice provider* before December 2, 2008, do not require MSW supervision (CMS, 2008). They were grandfathered in through hospice expertise and experience solely for that hospice organization.

Counseling is another core service in the Medicare Hospice Benefit to assist the patient and family in managing the stress and problems that arise at end of life. Counseling services must include the following three disciplines:

- **Spiritual care counselors**—Nondenominational spiritual care services are available to meet patient and family needs in accordance with their beliefs, customs, cultural background, religion, and desires. It is common for patients and families to struggle with or have questions about spiritual issues related to life closure. Through assessment and counseling, the spiritual counselor assists the patient and family to deal with these issues and hopefully find peace.

  The hospice spiritual counselor should facilitate visits by the patient's/family's local clergy, pastoral counselors, or other individuals who can support the patient's spiritual needs as necessary. If the patient and family do not have a connection to community spiritual care and desire support, the hospice spiritual counselor can provide that support. There are no federal hospice qualifications for a spiritual counselor, but state hospice licensure regulations or accreditation standards may have specific requirements (CMS, 2008).

- **Bereavement counselors**—Bereavement counseling is typically provided by the hospice to loved ones after the patient's death. Federal regulations require a minimum of 12 months of bereavement support after the patient dies, but NHPCO's Standards of Practice for Hospice Programs (2016) recommends that bereavement be provided for 13 months to support the family through the first anniversary of the patient's death. An initial bereavement assessment is completed at the start of care as part of the IDG's comprehensive assessment. This assessment can usually be completed by any member of the IDG, but usually the social worker or the spiritual counselor completes this assessment.

The hospice bereavement counselor serves as a core member of the IDG throughout the patient's service period and provides grief support to the family post patient death per their needs and desires. Bereavement counseling can be provided one-on-one (in person or phone) or in a group setting. Reimbursement for bereavement services is not provided by Medicare and most other payer sources, but it is a requirement for participation in the MHB. A bereavement counselor must be a qualified professional with experience or education in grief or loss counseling per the federal hospice qualifications (CMS, 2008).

- **Dietary counseling**—Hospices are required to assess the dietary needs of the patient and ensure that those needs are addressed by a qualified individual. If an RN can meet the patient's needs, then the RN can provide the dietary counseling. "If the needs of the patient exceed the expertise of the nurse, then the hospice must have available an appropriately trained and qualified individual, such as a registered dietitian or nutritionist, to meet the patient's dietary needs" (CMS, 2008, p. 41). The registered dietitian or nutritionist must meet the definition of an employee in the federal hospice CoPs and may not be contracted. Medicare provides the following definition (CMS, 2008, p. 118):

    *Employee means a person who: (1) works for the hospice and for whom the hospice is required to issue a W-2 form on his or her behalf; or (2) if the hospice is a subdivision of an agency or organization, an employee of the agency or organization who is assigned to the hospice; or (3) is a volunteer under the jurisdiction of the hospice.*

## HOSPICE "NONCORE" SERVICES

The hospice team members who are considered or referred to as noncore include hospice aides; pharmacists; speech, physical, and occupational therapists (as needed); homemakers; and volunteers. These services may be contracted by the hospice, but most hospice providers routinely employ hospice aides.

- **Hospice aide**—A hospice aide, working under the supervision of a registered nurse (RN), is an important part of the IDG. Aides tend to spend more time with the patient and the patient's family than the rest of the IDG. Because of this, they have a greater opportunity to develop relationships, learn valuable information that may not be communicated to other hospice team members, facilitate ongoing communication, and reinforce teaching with the patient and family. Hospice aides are assigned by an RN to assist a patient with:

  - Personal care (bathing, hair care, skin and nail care)
  - Activities of daily living (dressing, grooming, and more)
  - Toileting
  - Assistance in ambulation or exercises
  - Assistance in administration of medications that are ordinarily self-administered (per allowance of state law)

  Hospice aides follow an aide care plan that is specifically developed with the patient and family by the supervising RN. Aide activity is supervised minimally every 14 days by the supervising RN. The aide does not need to be present during the supervision visits per federal hospice regulations, but state hospice licensure regulations or accreditation standards may have specific requirements about this. An aide must also have a competency evaluation performed by an RN and must complete a minimum of 12 continuing education hours annually (CMS, 2008).

- **Homemaker**—Hospice providers must offer homemaker services per the federal hospice regulations. A qualified homemaker is an individual who (CMS, 2008):

- Can provide assistance in the maintenance of a safe and healthy environment and services to enable the individual to carry out the treatment plan

- Has successfully completed hospice orientation addressing the needs and concerns of patients and families coping with a terminal illness

- Can be a qualified hospice aide or a volunteer

- **Volunteers**—In the spirit of honoring that hospice care started as a volunteer movement, the Medicare Hospice Benefit mandated that volunteers continue to provide a key role in the provision of hospice care. The requirement for a volunteer force is unique to hospice. Volunteers are considered unpaid employees and must provide day-to-day administrative and/or direct patient care services in an amount that, at a minimum, equals 5% of the total patient care hours of all paid hospice employees and contract staff, including contract staff hours. The volunteer activities must be related to the hospice's administrative and direct patient care functions.

- **Pharmacists**—Most hospice providers contract with a pharmacy for the provision of patient medications and pharmacy services. The pharmacist is a valued and important part of the hospice team. Comprehensive medication therapy and management are critical in the control of symptoms in hospice and palliative care. Some of the functions a pharmacist performs include:

  - Assessing medication orders and drug profiles for appropriateness and timely provision of effective medications for symptom control

  - Serving as the designated dedicated individual for the review of patient medications and their related management

  - Educating and counseling the hospice team about medication therapy

  - Ensuring that patients and caregivers understand and adhere to the directions provided with medications

  - Participating in the review of the plan of care/IDG meetings as necessary

- **Therapists**—Therapy services such as physical, occupational, and speech language pathology are included in hospice. Services include training in the use of adaptive equipment, home safety assessment, and caregiver instruction toward use of good body mechanics for turning and lifting patients (CMS, 2008). Therapy for aggressive and routine rehabilitation is not a goal at end of life and would not be provided by hospice. Most hospice providers contract with individual therapists or a therapy agency, and services are provided to patients and families based on assessed patient/family needs.

# HOSPICE REIMBURSEMENT

Hospice is paid for through the Medicare Hospice Benefit, Medicaid Hospice Benefit, and many private insurers. If a person does not have coverage through Medicare, Medicaid, or a private insurance company, most hospice organizations work with the person in need and the family to ensure needed services can be provided. The following information addresses the most common payers.

## MEDICARE HOSPICE BENEFIT

The Medicare Hospice Benefit is covered under Medicare Part A (hospital insurance). Medicare beneficiaries who choose hospice care receive a full scope of medical and support services for their life-limiting illness. Hospice care also supports the family and loved ones through a variety of services. More than 90% of hospices in the United States are certified by Medicare. This is called "Medicare-certified." More than 80% of people who use hospice care are over the age of 65, and most are eligible for the services offered by the Medicare Hospice Benefit. This benefit covers all care related to the terminal prognosis that is determined medically necessary by the hospice physician. If there is a diagnosis that is not related to the terminal illness, the Medicare coverage the patient had before electing the hospice benefit covers this condition. In addition, most private health plans and Medicaid in 49 states and the District of Columbia cover hospice services. Medicaid coverage of hospice care mirrors Medicare coverage, but private health plan coverage can vary plan to plan. At this time, Oklahoma does not have a Medicaid Hospice Benefit.

## The Medicare Hospice Benefit: An Overview

Medicare is the largest healthcare payer for hospice in the United States. The Medicare Hospice Benefit was implemented in 1983 when the Health Care Financing Administration (HCFA), now called CMS, designed a comprehensive end-of-life benefit for Medicare beneficiaries. This was based on data and outcomes from a home healthcare hospice demonstration program funded by the National Cancer Institute from 1974 through 1977. In 1981, the Joint Commission on Accreditation of Hospitals received a grant from the W. K. Kellogg Foundation to research the phenomenon of hospice in the United States and to develop standards for hospice accreditation.

Congress created the Medicare Hospice Benefit, and it was implemented on November 1, 1983, with the inclusion of several cost-containment provisions. The hospice benefit includes capitations on the annual aggregate per patient expense and inpatient hospital utilization, thus promoting Medicare savings through the provision of home care services versus inpatient services (Davis, 1988).

Medicare regulations for hospices are located within the Code of Federal Regulations, Title §42, which is Public Health. Chapter 4 is titled "Centers for Medicare and Medicaid Services," and Part §418 is dedicated solely to hospice provision. Because these rules govern all Medicare-certified hospices, hospice team members should be familiar with the following subparts of the Medicare hospice regulations:

- Subpart A—General Provision and Definitions

  Contains general provisions of the hospice statute and definitions of specific terms that appear in the Conditions of Participation

- Subpart B—Eligibility, Election, and Duration of Benefits

  Contains requirements for hospice eligibility, certification, election of hospice, admission to hospice, revocation of the hospice benefit, change of hospice providers, and discharge

- Subpart C—Conditions of Participation—Patient Care

  Regulations that guide the delivery of patient care by the hospice IDG. Although all regulations in this section are important, patient rights, comprehensive assessment, care coordination and the plan of care, quality assessment performance improvement, and core service CoPs are critical for the delivery of quality of care. (Comprehensive assessment and plan of care are discussed more in Part 3.)

- Subpart D—Conditions of Participation: Organizational Environment

  Regulations that encompass how a hospice operates in relation to responsibility as the manager of hospice care; multiple locations; management of drugs and DME; hospice in contracted, inpatient, and nursing facilities; and personnel requirements

- Subpart F—Covered Services

  Includes services a hospice must cover and the requirements for coverage that affect payment

Appendixes A and B go into more detail about Subparts B and F. To become familiar and conversational about the details and specifics of the Medicare Hospice Benefit, read the Medicare hospice regulations.

## Related Versus Nonrelated Diagnoses

The Medicare Hospice Benefit is a *prognosis-based* benefit, which means that the patient must have a limited life expectancy and the hospice is responsible to care for and cover the costs for the terminal or primary diagnosis and all diagnoses that contribute to the terminal prognosis. The benefit covers services, drugs, supplies, and medical equipment related to the terminal diagnosis and all other diagnoses that contribute to the terminal prognosis.

"Cover" in this context generally means reimbursement or payment for appropriate hospice services. The Medicare Administrative Contractors (MACs) are the organizations that make payment determinations about coverage for hospice care. Hospice payment is predicated on law and regulations, and provider hospice organizations must understand and adhere to the rules. They can only pay for covered care. Where is covered care documented primarily? In the clinical record! Documentation is addressed in more depth in Part 2.

Medicare Part A (outside of the Medicare Health Benefit) covers services for diagnoses that do not contribute to the terminal prognosis (CMS, 1983). An example of this could be a patient with a primary terminal diagnosis of prostate cancer and a diagnosis of glaucoma. The glaucoma does not contribute to this patient's terminal prognosis. Determining relatedness is the responsibility of the hospice physician and can be a complex issue. NHPCO developed a process flowchart in 2014 to assist hospice physicians in making relatedness decisions, as shown in Figure 1.1.

The Conditions of Participation (CoPs) are the regulations that guide a hospice's provision of patient care and administrative processes. The only update to the 1983 hospice Conditions of Participation occurred in 2008. With that update, CMS focused the regulations on a patient-centered and outcome-oriented process that promotes the provision of quality patient care consistently for every patient. Compliance with regulations ensures that hospice providers meet requirements while monitoring and improving their own performance (CMS, 2008). CMS developed a core set of requirements for hospice services that incorporate the following:

- Patient rights
- Comprehensive assessment
- Patient care planning
- Coordination by a hospice IDG

The quality assessment and performance improvement (QAPI) program is an all-encompassing guide that enforces the idea that a provider's quality management system is the primary element to improved patient care performance (CMS, 2008).

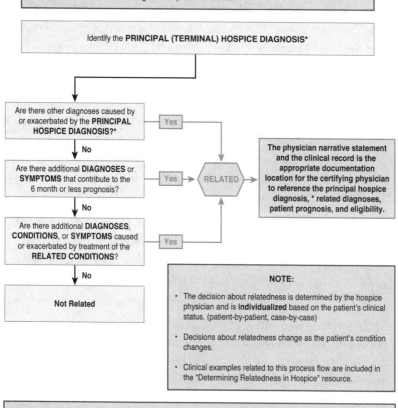

***Figure 1.1*** *Determining Relatedness to the Terminal Prognosis Process Flow*

© National Hospice and Palliative Care Organization, 2014. Reprinted with permission.

## COMPONENTS OF THE MEDICARE HOSPICE BENEFIT

The Medicare Hospice Benefit is complex, and the following are the most important tenets of this benefit.

### Eligibility

Individuals are eligible for the Medicare Hospice Benefit if they have Medicare Part A insurance and have been determined by the attending and the hospice physicians to have a terminal illness with a prognosis of 6 months or less if the illness follows its normal course (CMS, 1983). Eligibility is established by these physicians at the time of patient admission and then by a hospice physician continuously throughout the patient's length of stay. When a patient ceases to be eligible, meaning that the hospice physician no longer deems the patient is terminally ill with a limited prognosis of 6 months or less should the illness run its normal course, a hospice provider must discharge him or her from the hospice benefit (CMS, 2015a).

The MACs offer noncancer diagnosis guidelines, or local coverage determinations (LCDs), to assist physicians in determining eligibility for hospice service. Although these guidelines provide clinical criteria for a variety of noncancer diseases, it is the hospice physician's medical judgment that ultimately determines eligibility.

Demonstrating eligibility in clinical documentation is an ongoing process for hospice organizations. It should be evidenced/apparent at the time of admission to hospice and in the initial certification and recertification by the hospice physician. It is also the responsibility of the interdisciplinary group members to evidence eligibility throughout the service period in their clinical documentation. In the past several years, CMS has increased scrutiny around eligibility and has increased regulations centering on the certification process to ensure providers are admitting and providing services to hospice-eligible and appropriate patients only.

### Hospice Election

Hospice care is available for a beneficiary in two 90-day periods followed by an unlimited number of 60-day periods as long as the patient remains eligible for hospice per the Medicare requirements. A patient who chooses hospice care must sign an "election of hospice" statement. The patient's/representative's signature on the hospice election statement is the trigger to begin hospice services and includes language that the patient acknowledges that hospice provides a palliative approach to care versus a curative one. It is important to note that verbal election of hospice services is not allowed, and services may not begin until a signature on the election is obtained by the hospice provider. When individuals elect the Medicare Hospice Benefit, they waive the right to Medicare payment for other services related to the terminal prognosis (CMS, 2005).

As of October 1, 2014, hospice providers are required to file the hospice Notice of Election (NOE) with their MAC to properly enforce this waiver and prevent payments to nonhospice providers during the time of hospice service. The NOE must be filed within 5 calendar days after the effective date of hospice election. The effective date of the hospice election is the same as the hospice admission date. A timely filed NOE is one that is submitted to, and accepted by, the MAC within 5 calendar days after the patient's hospice election. When an NOE is not filed in a timely manner, Medicare does not reimburse the provider for the days of hospice care from the hospice admission date to the date the NOE is submitted to, and accepted by, the MAC. These days are deemed provider-liable, and the provider may not bill Medicare or the patient for these days (CMS, 2015a).

According to CMS, the election of hospice statement must contain the following content to be valid. Hospice providers or organizations may design their own election form, but these seven elements must be present:

1. Identification of the particular hospice that will provide care to the individual.

2. The individual's or representative's (as applicable) acknowledgment that the individual has been given a full understanding of hospice care, particularly the **palliative versus the curative** nature of treatment.

3. The individual's or representative's (as applicable) acknowledgment that the individual understands that certain Medicare services are waived by the election.

4. The effective date of the election, which may be the first day of hospice care or a later date, but may be no earlier than the date of the election statement. An individual may not designate an effective date that is retroactive.

5. The individual's designated attending physician (if any). Information identifying the attending physician recorded on the election statement should provide enough detail so that it is clear which physician or nurse practitioner (NP) was designated as the attending physician. This information should include information that clearly identifies the attending physician.

6. The individual's acknowledgment that the designated attending physician was the individual's or the representative's choice.

7. The signature of the individual or representative (CMS, 2015a).

## Certification of Terminal Illness

An individual must be certified as terminally ill by a physician to receive hospice care services. Benefit periods are administered as follows:

1. Two 90-day benefit periods.

2. Unlimited 60-day benefit periods as long as the patient remains hospice-eligible. For the first 90-day benefit period, the patient's chosen attending physician and the hospice physician complete a certification of terminal illness form including a statement that the patient has a 6-month-or-less prognosis. A certification of terminal illness is completed by only one physician (usually the hospice physician) for subsequent hospice benefit periods. If a patient remains hospice-eligible past the first two 90-day benefit periods, a physician or nurse practitioner is required to complete a face-to-face visit with the patient to assess and validate continuing eligibility **prior to each subsequent certification period** (CMS, 2015a). It is critical for a hospice to ensure their process for certification of terminal illness is accurate, or they risk not being paid for all days in that particular benefit period. Providers should have a procedure in place to review all certifications for timing, content, and quality (medical necessity, care, appropriateness).

3. Timing of the certification. For each benefit period of hospice coverage, the hospice must obtain a written certification of terminal illness by the hospice physician and the individual's attending physician (if it is the first 90-day benefit period) no later than 2 calendar days after hospice care is initiated (by the end of the third day). If the written certification is not obtained, a verbal or oral certification must be obtained in that same time frame.

4. Verbal certification from the physician stating that the patient is terminally ill, with a prognosis of 6 months or less. The verbal certification is documented in the clinical record by the hospice staff member receiving it and should be easily identifiable. This documentation does not require the physician's signature. Certifications for a benefit period may be completed up to 15 days before hospice care is elected or the new benefit period begins. Certifications of terminal illness are required for every benefit period, and the written certification must be obtained prior to submission of a claim to the hospice provider's MAC (CMS, 2015a).

5. Physician narrative statement. The physician's narrative explanation of the clinical findings that support a life expectancy of 6 months or less has been a requirement of the certification/recertification process since 2009. In the first 90-day benefit period, either the attending or a hospice physician completes the narrative statement. Because the hospice physician has extensive experience in determining eligibility, it is recommended that he/she complete this narrative statement. The narrative may be a part of the certification/recertification form or an addendum and must include an "attestation" statement. This attestation statement validates that the certifying physician composed the narrative statement and is addressed in the information that follows:

   a. If the narrative is a part of the certification form, then it must be inserted immediately above the physician's signature.

   b. If it is an addendum to the certification or recertification form, the physician must also sign immediately following the narrative.

    c. The narrative must appear directly above the physician signature attesting that, by signing, the physician confirms that he/she composed this patient-specific narrative based on his/her review of the patient's medical record or, if applicable, his or her examination of the patient (CMS, 2015a).

    d. The narrative statement:

      i. May be dictated

      ii. Must reflect the patient's individual clinical circumstances

      iii. May not contain check boxes or standard language used for all patients (for example, not a form)

    e. Content of the narrative statement should include:

      i. Clinical factors associated with a patient's prognosis < 6 months

      ii. Patient history as relevant to the prognosis and individual clinical circumstances

      iii. Relevant hospitalizations or emergency department visits

      iv. Evidence of disease progression

      v. Trajectory of patient decline

      vi. Symptoms indicating progression or severity

      vii. Prognostic signs noted on comprehensive assessment

      viii. Lab or X-ray data (as applicable)

      ix. Reference to LCDs

      x. Other LCD factors

      xi. Lack of LCD factors

      xii. Other data that supports medical necessity based on the patient's/family's unique condition and circumstances

6. Hospice face-to-face encounter (F2F). A face-to-face encounter is an in-person patient visit by a hospice physician or nurse practitioner to assess the patient for continuing hospice eligibility. The physician or NP must have the face-to-face encounter with each hospice patient prior to the beginning of the patient's third benefit

period and prior to each subsequent benefit period. The face-to-face encounter is compliant when the following criteria are met:

a. Timing—The encounter must be completed prior to the recertification for the third benefit period and each subsequent benefit period thereafter. The visit must occur no more than 30 calendar days before the start of the third hospice benefit period recertification and each subsequent recertification, and it is considered timely if it occurs on the first day of the benefit period.

b. Attestation requirements—A hospice physician or nurse practitioner who performs the face-to-face encounter must attest in writing that he or she had a face-to-face encounter with the patient, including the date of the encounter. The attestation, its accompanying signature, and the date signed must be a separate and distinct section of, or an addendum to, the recertification form, and it must be clearly titled as the "Face-to-Face Attestation." If a nurse practitioner or noncertifying hospice physician performed the face-to-face encounter, the attestation must state that the clinical findings of that visit were provided to the certifying physician, for use in determining whether the patient continues to have a life expectancy of 6 months or less, should the illness run its normal course.

c. Missed or late face-to-face encounter—When the face-to-face encounter is missed, or completed late, the patient ceases to be eligible for the Medicare Hospice Benefit. In this instance, a hospice provider discharges the patient from the Medicare Hospice Benefit and continues to provide care for the patient at its own expense until the face-to-face encounter is completed. The hospice can then readmit the patient to the Medicare Hospice Benefit, which re-establishes Medicare eligibility. The readmission should be treated as a new admission to the Medicare Hospice Benefit, which requires the patient/representative to sign a new hospice election statement and the hospice provider to file the NOE into Common Working File (CWF) within 5 calendar days after the hospice election (CMS, 2015b).

d. Physicians and NPs—A hospice physician or a hospice nurse practitioner can complete the encounter. A hospice physician can be employed by the hospice or working under contract with the hospice. A hospice nurse practitioner must be an employee of the hospice. (Definition of employee per the Medicare hospice CoPs: A hospice employee is one who receives a W-2 from the hospice or who volunteers for the hospice. If the hospice is a subdivision of an agency or organization, an employee of that agency or organization assigned to the hospice is also considered a hospice employee.)

> **NOTE** Physician assistants (PAs), clinical nurse specialists, and outside attending physicians are not authorized to perform the face-to-face encounter for hospice recertification purposes.

e. Exceptional circumstances—Exceptional circumstances may prevent the completion of a face-to-face encounter prior to the start of the benefit period. For example, if the patient is admitted over a weekend in an emergency situation, it may be impossible for a hospice physician or nurse practitioner to see the patient until the following Monday. Or if CMS data systems are unavailable, the hospice may be unaware that the patient is in the third benefit period. A F2F encounter that occurs within 2 days after admission will be considered to be timely when there is documentation of an exceptional circumstance noted and explained in the patient's clinical record. If the patient dies within 2 days of admission without a face-to-face encounter, a face-to-face encounter is considered complete (CMS, 2015b).

Table 1.1 includes the content required for a valid certification of terminal illness.

**TABLE 1.1** Certifying a Terminal Illness

| | 1st 90-day period | 2nd 90-day period | 1st and subsequent 60-day periods |
|---|---|---|---|
| **Verbal certification** | ☑ If written certification is not obtained within 2 days of the start of care date<br><br>☑ No physician signature required | ☑ If written certification is not obtained within 2 days of the start of care date<br><br>☑ No physician signature required | ☑ If written certification is not obtained within 2 days of the start of care date<br><br>☑ No physician signature required |
| **Written certification form** | ☑ Signed by attending physician and hospice medical director/ hospice physician<br><br>☑ Physician signature and date required | ☑ Signed by hospice medical director/ hospice physician<br><br>☑ Physician signature and date required | ☑ Signed by hospice medical director/ hospice physician<br><br>☑ Physician signature and date required |
| **Face-to-face encounter attestation statement** | | | ☑ Face-to-face encounter attestation statement<br><br>☑ Physician/ NP signature and date required below attestation |
| **Physician narrative statement and attestation statement** | ☑ Narrative statement<br><br>☑ Attestation statement<br><br>☑ Physician signature required below attestation | ☑ Narrative statement<br><br>☑ Attestation statement<br><br>☑ Physician signature required below attestation | ☑ Narrative statement<br><br>☑ Attestation statement<br><br>☑ Physician signature required below attestation |

Table from NHPCO. ©2013 Reprinted with permission.

# REVOCATION/CHANGE OF PROVIDER/DISCHARGE

The primary reason for discharge from hospice is death; however, patients may have circumstances that require a discharge for other reasons.

## REVOCATION OF THE MEDICARE HOSPICE BENEFIT— THE PATIENT'S RIGHT TO REVOCATION

Patients may revoke their hospice benefits at any time and for any reason. This is important to note because only the hospice patient/beneficiary can revoke his/her benefit; hospice organizations may not revoke the Medicare Hospice Benefit. When patients revoke hospice, they return to the Medicare coverage they had before electing the hospice benefit. Should they choose, the patient can re-elect hospice at any time.

Revocation is a patient right, and only a patient (or the patient's representative) can revoke hospice benefits. A revocation is effective on the date the patient (or the patient's representative) signs the hospice revocation form. A revocation can never be backdated, and it must be in writing. Verbal revocation is never valid under the Medicare Hospice Benefit. Hospice providers should document as much detail as possible related to the patient's reason for the revocation as well as discussion about the patient's right to return to hospice care at any time in the future (CMS, 2005).

There is no such thing as an "automatic" revocation of a patient's hospice benefit, such as if the patient seeks emergent care related to the terminal prognosis or does not comply with the plan of care. Again, revocation of the hospice benefit is a patient right that can only be executed by the patient (or the patient's representative).

## CHANGE OF HOSPICE PROVIDER— ANOTHER PATIENT RIGHT

Another right of the patient under the Medicare Hospice Benefit is the ability to change or transfer hospice providers once per benefit period. The patient can choose to transfer from one provider to another for any reason and without a break in service. The patient remains in the same benefit period, and continuity of all hospice services under the individualized plan of care continues. To change hospice providers, the patient (or the representative) files a signed statement with the current hospice and with the newly designated hospice that indicates the effective date of the transfer and the to/from hospice provider information (CMS, 2005).

## DISCHARGE FROM HOSPICE

A patient can be discharged from hospice service, but the allowable reasons are limited as follows:

- The beneficiary dies.

- The patient moves out of the hospice organization's geographic area or enters a facility where the hospice does not have a contract for service.

- If at any time the hospice physician determines, in his or her medical opinion, that the patient no longer has a 6-month or less prognosis and is no longer terminally ill, the hospice is required by regulation to discharge the patient from service.

- The hospice may discharge a patient in extraordinary circumstances related to its inability to continue to provide hospice care. These circumstances could be related to compromised patient or hospice staff safety. For example, if the patient's (or another person(s) in the patient's home) "behavior is disruptive, abusive, or uncooperative to the extent that delivery of care to the patient or the ability of the hospice to operate effectively is seriously impaired, the hospice can consider discharge for cause" (CMS, 2015b, p. 14). There must be comprehensive documentation in the clinical record that the hospice team attempted to resolve the problem without success and that the last option was to discharge for cause. Documentation in such an instance should include:
    - Discussion with the patient and family that a discharge for cause is being considered
    - Interventions implemented to resolve the problem(s) presented by the patient's behavior or situation

- Notice of discharge for cause to the patient/family, the state survey agency, and the provider's MAC (CMS, 2015b)
- The hospice provider must also obtain a discharge order from the hospice physician, document consultation with the patient's attending physician about the discharge, and provide/document a discharge plan to the patient.

# THE FOUR LEVELS OF HOSPICE CARE

There are four levels of patient care under the Medicare Hospice Benefit, and every Medicare-certified hospice must have the ability to provide every level.

1. **Routine home care (RHC)**—Most patients in hospice receive care at this level in the place they call home (private residence, assisted living facility (ALF), nursing home, and so on). Care provision from the hospice team is intermittent (visits), and the frequency of services is determined by the patient's and family's assessed needs. If the patient requires hourly care and support that a caregiver cannot provide, the hospice team can assist the patient and family to determine options for required care. However, hourly care in the home for a patient whose disease symptoms are well controlled is not covered by Medicare (CMS, 2015b).

2. **Inpatient respite care**—This level of care is short-term inpatient care to provide respite for the person(s) caring for the patient in the home when they need a break or relief from that patient care. Respite may be provided occasionally and for no more than 5 consecutive days at a time in a Medicare-certified nursing facility, hospital, or hospice inpatient facility.

   Respite care cannot be provided in an assisted living facility or non-Medicare-certified hospice house. While the patient is inpatient for respite care, the hospice team provides continued services per the patient's plan of care. Coordination between the hospice team and the facility staff is critical to maintaining the patient's quality of care. The hospice team is the manager of the patient's plan of care during respite care, and the facility staff should not make changes in care without consulting the hospice first (CMS, 2015b).

 **NOTE** Respite may not be provided to hospice patients who reside in a facility (such as a long-term care nursing facility).

3. **General inpatient care (GIP)**—If a patient experiences a medical crisis and the symptoms cannot be managed in the home (or other residence), he or she can be transitioned to GIP care for 24/7 intense attention. This level of care can be provided in a Medicare-certified hospital, skilled nursing facility, or hospice inpatient facility. GIP may be needed when the patient's medical condition requires a short-term inpatient stay for pain control or acute symptom management that cannot feasibly be provided in other settings. There must be acuity of the patient's symptoms and intensity of hospice interventions to justify a GIP day. Examples of appropriate GIP care could include:

   - Pain or symptom crisis

   - Intractable nausea/vomiting

   - Unmanageable respiratory distress

   - Sudden decline necessitating intensive nursing intervention

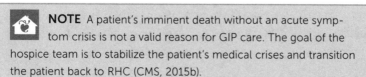 **NOTE** A patient's imminent death without an acute symptom crisis is not a valid reason for GIP care. The goal of the hospice team is to stabilize the patient's medical crises and transition the patient back to RHC (CMS, 2015b).

4. **Continuous home care (CHC)**—CHC is hourly care that is provided during a period of medical crisis to maintain an individual at home (or other residence). A patient who qualifies for CHC requires continuous care when the medical condition necessitates a short-term inpatient intervention for pain control or acute symptom management that requires predominantly nursing care to manage acute medical symptoms. A minimum of 8 hours of

nursing, hospice aide, or homemaker care must be provided to the patient during a 24-hour day, which begins and ends at midnight, and the services provided must be predominantly nursing care, provided by an RN, an LPN, or an LVN.

CHC does not need to be continuous, meaning that the minimum 8 hours does not need to be provided in a row. A nurse may provide 5 hours of care in the morning and a hospice aide may provide 3 hours of care later the same day. Like the GIP level of care, there must be acuity of the patient's symptoms and intensity of hospice interventions to justify a CHC day. This level of care can be provided to a patient who resides in a long-term care facility. However, Medicare regulations do not permit CHC to be provided in an inpatient facility (a hospice inpatient unit, a hospital, or SNF) (CMS, 2015b).

# MEDICARE HOSPICE QUALITY: WHAT IS IT?

Quality in hospice is multidimensional and includes many regulations and care considerations. With the 2008 update to the CoPs, CMS included a comprehensive CoP dedicated to quality assessment and performance improvement. The purpose of the QAPI CoP is to set a clear expectation that hospices must demonstrate a proactive approach to improve their performance and focus on improved patient/family care and activities that impact patient health and safety.

CMS stresses the improvement in systems to improve processes and patient outcomes. The regulation requires a hospice to develop, implement, and maintain an effective, ongoing, hospice-wide data-driven QAPI program. The hospice's governing body must oversee the program and ensure that the program:

- Reflects the complexity of its organization and services
- Involves all hospice services (including those services furnished under contract or arrangement)

- Focuses on indicators related to improved palliative outcomes
- Takes actions to demonstrate improvement in hospice performance

The hospice must be able to evidence a fully functional QAPI program in writing and be able to demonstrate its operation to CMS (CMS, 2008).

§418.58 Condition of Participation: Quality Assessment and Performance Improvement (QAPI) defines the components of a compliant QAPI program including:

- Program scope
- Program data
- Program activities
- Performance improvement projects
- Executive responsibilities

The hospice must complete a system-wide self-assessment and identify areas for improvement. Methods the hospice uses for the self-assessment are flexible and could include:

- A review of current documentation (for example, review of clinical records, incident reports, complaints, and patient satisfaction surveys)
- Patient care
- Direct observation of clinical performance and operating systems
- Interviews with patients or staff (CMS, 2008)

The information collected should be based on criteria or measures generated by the medical and professional/technical staff and reflect hospice best practice patterns, staff performance, and patient outcomes (CMS, 2008).

Although the structure of the plan is at a hospice provider's discretion, the following elements should be included:

- Program objectives
- All patient care disciplines

- Description of how the program will be administered and coordinated
- Methodology for monitoring and evaluating the quality of care
- Priorities for resolution of problems
- Monitoring to determine effectiveness of action
- Oversight responsibility reports to governing body
- Documentation of the review of its own QAPI program (CMS, 2008)

## HOSPICE QUALITY REPORTING TO CMS: LINKING QUALITY TO PAYMENT

Hospice providers began submitting quality measures because of provisions in the FY2014 final Hospice Wage Index rule. Hospice providers are required to collect and submit an admission and discharge Hospice Item Set (HIS) for each patient admission to hospice, regardless of payer or patient age. The HIS is a standardized set of items intended to capture patient-level data.

The goal for CMS is to add quality measures to the HIS in subsequent rulemaking and implement public reporting for hospice providers (CMS, 2013). The FY2016 final Hospice Wage Index rule established submission thresholds for HIS data with a 2018 target goal of 90% submission within the 30-day submission time frame for the year or face a 1% point reduction to the market basket percentage increase for that fiscal year (CMS, 2015a).

CMS online resources for QAPI and quality:

- Hospice Item Set (HIS) (https://www.cms.gov/Medicare/ Quality-Initiatives-Patient-Assessment-Instruments/ Hospice-Quality-Reporting/Hospice-Item-Set-HIS.html)
- HIS Technical Information (https://www.cms.gov/Medicare/ Quality-Initiatives-Patient-Assessment-Instruments/ Hospice-Quality-Reporting/HIS-Technical-Information.html)

- Guidance Manual for Completion of the Hospice Item Set (HIS) (https://www.cms.gov/Medicare/Quality-Initiatives-Patient-Assessment-Instruments/Hospice-Quality-Reporting/Downloads/HIS-Manual.pdf)
- Getting Started with Hospice Item Set (HIS) Reporting: Checklist and Quick Tips (https://www.cms.gov/Medicare/Quality-Initiatives-Patient-Assessment-Instruments/Hospice-Quality-Reporting/Downloads/Fact-Sheet-Getting-Started-with-the-HIS---Checklist-and-Quick-Tips.pdf)
- Data Submission Requirements Under the Hospice Quality Reporting Program (https://www.ecfr.gov/cgi-bin/text-idx?SID=1489973fe3a92e8e03c3e9f76550cef7&mc=true&node=se42.3.418_1312&rgn=div8)

## CONSUMER ASSESSMENT OF HEALTHCARE PROVIDERS AND SYSTEMS (CAHPS) HOSPICE SURVEY

Another tenet of quality is feedback, and it is used in QAPI. Medicare-certified hospices must also submit CAHPS data to the Hospice CAHPS Data Center via a contracted CMS-approved vendor who collects the CAHPS Hospice Survey data on the hospice's behalf. The CAHPS Hospice Survey measures and assesses the experiences of patients who died while receiving hospice care, as well as the experiences of their family or other primary caregivers. The standardized CAHPS Hospice Survey instrument is composed of the following measures:

- Hospice team communication
- Timely care
- Respect for family members
- Emotional support
- Support for religious and spiritual beliefs
- Help for symptoms
- Information continuity
- Side effects of pain medication
- Hospice care training

The definition of "survey of individual patients" is a collection of data from at least 600 individual patients selected by statistical sampling methods. If a hospice provider's total, annual, unique, survey-eligible, deceased patient count for the prior calendar year is fewer than 50 patients, the hospice is eligible for an exemption from submitting CAHPS data in the current calendar year. To qualify for this exemption, the hospice must submit to CMS its total, annual, unique, survey-eligible, deceased patient count for the prior calendar year. Failure to submit required data shall result in a 2% point reduction to the market basket percentage increase for that fiscal year (CMS, 2013). You can obtain information on the CAHPS Hospice Survey at http://www.hospicecahpssurvey.org.

## CMS HOSPICE COMPARE—THE PUBLIC DISPLAY OF QUALITY MEASURES AND OTHER HOSPICE DATA

CMS is developing the infrastructure for hospice public reporting, which is a requirement of the Affordable Care Act. The CMS Hospice Compare website provides valuable information regarding the quality of care provided by Medicare-certified hospice agencies throughout the nation. Consumers can search for all Medicare-approved hospice providers that serve their city or zip code (which would include the quality measures and CAHPS Hospice Survey results) and then find the agencies offering the types of services they need, along with provider quality information (CMS, 2016).

CMS makes quality measure data available to individual hospice providers prior to publicly reporting information about the quality of care. These "preview reports," which contain quality measure data, are made available in CMS's system prior to public reporting and offer providers the opportunity to review and correct their quality measure data prior to public reporting on the CMS Hospice Compare website for hospice agencies (CMS, 2016). CMS implemented the CMS Hospice Compare website in 2017.

# DEFINING HOSPICE NURSING

Whatever the organizational structure of the hospice, the hospice nurse plays a key role on the team. Hospice care practice is the provision of palliative care for the terminally ill and their families, with the emphasis on their physical, psychosocial, emotional, and spiritual needs (Rome, Luminais, Bourgeois, & Blais, 2011). Hospice care is a synthesis of special skills that are used to create the environment for the best outcomes for hospice patients and their families.

The hospice nurse's role is often that of case or care manager as the nurse coordinates the implementation of the plan of care. Whatever the role defined by the organization, the following are key aspects of the hospice care specialty that must be learned, nurtured, and improved through continued education and experience. Experienced clinicians new to hospice may be paired with an experienced hospice nurse as a preceptor through the new clinician's orientation. As with any specialty, home healthcare clinicians require additional orientation, education, and experience to successfully make the transition to hospice. Hospice is very different from home healthcare practice even though some of the care interventions appear similar, and the care site, the patient's home, may be the same.

Hospice is a unique niche in healthcare, and many nurses who practice in its realm say it is also a calling. Hospice nursing requires specialty clinical skills related to end-of-life issues, but also compassion, excellent listening skills, and the ability to work as part of a close-knit team. The hospice nurse is the first person of the hospice team to physically assess the patient, develop the initial plan of care, and ultimately manage that plan of care. The hospice nurse works in tandem with the rest of the interdisciplinary group to coordinate care and move the patient toward measurable goals. No matter the level of experience a nurse has in joining a hospice organization, the hospice organization must nurture each nurse with a comprehensive orientation, peer support, preceptorships (as needed), and continuing education.

## HALLMARKS OF EFFECTIVE HOSPICE CARE

Hospice care workers must possess a wide variety of skills—some that are unique to the hospice care field, which might require learning new skills or a period of adaptation. The following sections provide an introduction.

### Pain and Symptom Management Skills

This is a specialty area in hospice. Because of the teamwork in hospice, this is often an interdisciplinary effort with input from the hospice nurse, the physician, the pharmacist, and other team members, such as a social worker and a spiritual counselor. Because the focus of care is palliative and supportive, it is imperative that hospice nurses be competent in pain assessment, intervention, and evaluation. The fifth vital sign, pain, should be assessed during every patient encounter. Modalities for pain relief and optimal comfort range from pharmaceutical agents to acupuncture, imagery, massage, and other care interventions. Many patients receive a complement of pain solutions (pharmacologic and nonpharmacologic).

### Knowledge and Concepts Related to Death and Dying

The hospice philosophy of care views death as a natural part of life. Dame Cicely Saunders's development of the total pain theory and hospice approach as well as Dr. Elizabeth Kübler-Ross's research on the stages of dying serve as theoretical guideposts for hospice teams. Hospice teams need to understand the concepts that are the hallmarks of hospice and integrate them into their critical thinking skills, evidence-based practice, and care delivery at end of life.

### Stress Management

Hospice teams have varied mechanisms for supporting themselves and each other. Hospice care may be stressful for clinicians and other hospice workers. Team and team member support may be informal, such as debriefing with another team member, or structured, such as scheduled meetings with a trained facilitator. It is important that all hospice team members take care of themselves and find activities and events that promote emotional well-being and nurture and support growth and healing.

Whatever model staff support takes, it is a means for sharing, caring, team building, validating, and processing the important work of hospice.

## Active Listening Skills

Communication skills are essential for effective hospice team members. There is untold intimacy and poignancy in hospice. A clinician walks into the homes of patients who may have been battling cancer for years and are now ready to change the focus from fighting the disease to making the best of their last days in their chosen way. The patient's sole priority may be symptom management, or it may be the well-being of a pet or the maintenance of a garden. These values also become the hospice team's priorities to support care and respect the patient's wishes. The psychosocial and spiritual components of hospice are important to the patient's quality of life and the overall patient/family experience. The hospice team can facilitate closure or the mending of difficult relationships.

Communication skills include active listening, realizing the work of "getting things in order," presence as an intervention, and being sensitively cued to what the patient and family are saying (and sometimes asking for). An example is Sarah, a 39-year-old woman with an aggressive, recurrent breast cancer. At a nursing visit, Sarah said to the hospice nurse, "I want to renew my vows with my husband before I die." The nurse said she would "talk to her later" because she was doing the patient's dressing change; however, this discussion did not occur. Sarah later expressed the same wish to the HHA, who reported it at the patient care conference. Because of this team effort, Sarah did renew her vows before her death. Especially in hospice, because of the limited time factor, patient and family needs must be addressed in a timely manner. In addition, this example shows an important component of hospice: spiritual care.

Patient and family needs, both those clearly articulated and those that are more veiled, should be identified to ensure that the hospice team is addressing and meeting those needs. Spiritual and other psychosocial needs are a key component in the provision of high-quality hospice nursing.

## Sense of Humor

It has only been in the past few years that the healing power of laughter has finally come to be recognized. A sense of humor helps the entire team, the patients, and their families on particularly rough days or in meeting unique challenges.

## Flexibility

Patients and families in hospice control their care and care planning. Because the days shared with the hospice team are the patient's last, the patient calls the shots. This includes scheduling, visit times, length of visits, and a myriad of other decisions. Respect for and acceptance of the patient's choices and decisions are part of effective daily operations in hospice and are required by law through patient self-determination acts.

## Hospice and Palliative Care Knowledge

It is important that the hospice team members have a strong base of knowledge grounded in hospice care and practice. There is a large body of literature related to hospice and the many aspects of end-of-life care. Additionally, families need accurate and thorough information to help their loved one. Hospice team members should provide as much information as the patient and family choose to receive. "When is he/she going to die?" is a common and justifiable concern. The Signs and Symptoms of Approaching Death sidebar provides a useful list of some of the signs that family members may expect to see with the approach of death.

## The Customer Service Experience and Feedback for QAPI

In the best healthcare, regardless of setting, there should be continual efforts toward quality improvement. This may include how to better serve customers/patients; how to better identify, document and track, and trend infections; and other examples. The comments and feedback gleaned from a number of sources can assist in improving care and processes.

## SIGNS AND SYMPTOMS OF APPROACHING DEATH

The following are some of the signs and symptoms as death approaches. Some symptoms may not appear, and the symptoms will not all appear at the same time. Some of the most common symptoms are:

- **Cooling of the extremities**—The patient's hands, arms, or feet are cool to the touch, and mottling or a purplish coloring may appear. Sometimes the skin also darkens, appears pale, bluish, or yellowish with the decrease in circulation as death approaches. Interventions are related to keeping the patient warm, but electric blankets should not be used for safety reasons.

- **Breathing slows and becomes irregular**—Cheyne-Stokes breathing may occur as the cerebrum, the control center for respirations, begins to fail. This breathing is usually characterized by irregularity and apnea, sometimes with long periods between breaths.

- **The patient sleeps almost all the time**—This occurs as the slow but progressive failure of body systems occurs and metabolic needs decrease proportionately toward death.

- **Fluids begin to build up in some patients**—This may appear as increased secretions in the throat or a sound like a "rattle." The body can no longer absorb the secretions, and the fluid is heard as a result. The rattle, which can be distressing to family members, can sometimes be controlled with medication. The patient may also be suctioned or repositioned for comfort in some instances.

- **The patient may appear confused or restless**—Confusion is a common part of the death process and may be very upsetting to family members. Caregiver and family members may want to reassure the patient or provide presence to the patient. It is important that the restlessness be assessed as being caused by the lack of oxygenation and not from pain or other discomfort.

*(continues)*

*(continued)*

> No matter what the symptoms or signs of approaching death, it is important that family members support the patient through this changing period with their presence and support. *Patients can still hear* even if their eyes appear glassy and unresponsive.

## DIFFERENCES IN GOALS BETWEEN HOME HEALTH AND HOSPICE NURSING

The goals for care in hospice are different from those in home healthcare. Although goals in hospice must be measurable, they are focused toward achieving comfort, control, quality of life, and peaceful life closure. For example, wound care in hospice may not necessarily have a goal of healing, but rather maintaining comfort, managing odor, and preventing pain and/or further tissue damage if possible.

## SKILLS AND KNOWLEDGE NEEDED FOR HOSPICE CARE

The following are some of the core resources and areas of knowledge that provide the foundational information to be successful in hospice. Like other practice areas, managers and clinicians must stay up to date with changing regulatory requirements.

The Medicare hospice regulations, including:

- Subpart A—General Provision and Definitions
- Subpart B—Eligibility, Election, and Duration of Benefits
- Subpart C—Conditions of Participation—Patient Care
- Subpart D—Conditions of Participation: Organizational Environment
- Subpart F—Covered Services

Familiarity with state hospice licensure regulations, the NHPCO Standards of Practice for Hospice Programs, and accreditation organization standards (as applicable) is also recommended. Currently, three accreditation organizations are approved by CMS for hospice:

- The Joint Commission (TJC) (jointcommission.org)
- Community Health Accreditation Partner (CHAP) (chapinc.org)
- Accreditation Commission for Health Care (ACHC) (achc.org)

From a clinical perspective, hospice nurses must possess excellent assessment skills, pain and symptom management knowledge, critical thinking skills, and the ability to see the patient holistically. In addition, the hospice nurse should have:

- A repertoire of service-driven and patient-oriented interpersonal skills

  Community liaison and public relations activities are part of the hospice nurse's busy day. The nurse is representing hospice, so it's important to make those impressions positive.

- The ability to pay incredible attention to detail

  This is true both in addressing complex patient and family care needs and in documentation. Both are equally important in the provision of high-quality care.

- The possession of multifaceted skills accompanied by flexibility

  It is the hospice team member that must "bend" or renegotiate to meet patient and family needs and achieve patient-centered outcomes. This flexibility usually includes visiting times and scheduling but can also include aspects that center on accommodating patient and family/caregiver needs.

- The possession of a reliable car and safe, effective driving skills

  The hospice team member in the community must like, or at least not mind, driving (even in inclement weather) and have a good sense of direction.

- The ability to assume responsibility for the patient and family's care and the patient's plan of care

  Holistic care is a reality in quality hospice care. From the initial hospice assessment through the identification of patient and family needs and challenges, the hospice nurse assumes the planning and follow-through for care. Sometimes only a limited number of core hospice team members are involved in the care, depending on the patient and family needs. Because of these factors, the hospice nurse in the community setting can directly affect the care and see the results of that planned and continually evaluated care. Close communication is required between the hospice nurse and the other team members and any case managers involved with the care. This patient-management function, with its associated prioritizing and sometimes complex decision-making, makes hospice practice unique. It is from this aspect that hospice team members often receive personal satisfaction and positive feedback from patients and their families, friends, and caregivers.

- Strong clinical skills and the ability to function as both a specialist and a generalist clinician

  Hospice patients may be from all age groups, from infants to the elderly. The diagnoses and care needs of patients may vary from day to day. Within the hospice organization, a wide range of clinical problems and nursing diagnoses may exist. Developing an area of expertise and acting as a resource for clinicians new to hospice care are important assets for the individual clinician or manager's own professional growth.

- Self-direction and the ability to function autonomously in a non-structured environment

  Self-direction means having well-developed and effective time-management skills to address the many aspects of care, including scheduled visits, documentation, and detail-oriented administrative duties (for example, completing and updating plans of care, returning a phone call in a timely way).

- The desire to continue learning and being open to new information and clinical skills

  This is particularly important given the many new kinds of technologies being used in the home setting. New pain and symptom management methods and ethical dilemmas may be some of the care problems competent clinicians and managers address daily.

- A sincere appreciation of people

  This includes interacting positively with and being empathetic to all patients, families, and caregivers, who are often in the midst of crises. Hospice team members use their observation, assessment, teaching, and training skills to maintain patient safety in the home. This teaching or consulting role brings job satisfaction as well as comfort and security to the families.

- The ability to be open and sincerely accepting of people's unique and chosen lifestyles and of the effects that these lifestyles have on their health

  Being accepting is easier said than done! Every nurse has cared for patients with end-stage COPD who continue to smoke and do not adhere to the safety instructions they have been taught regarding oxygen. These ethical dilemmas of safety versus self-determination are a part of professional hospice practice.

- The awareness and acceptance that a constant balance must be maintained between clinical and administrative demands

  The clinician must know that both demands are equally important, but in different ways and for different reasons.

- An acceptance of change

  It is important to expect that things will constantly change. Regulations, mergers/acquisitions, documentation systems, reimbursement mechanisms, and many other facets of healthcare change so frequently that it is a challenge to keep up. Embracing change helps ease the stress associated with the change process.

- Knowledge of the economics of healthcare and the larger environment that is affecting hospice

  The basic knowledge of reimbursement, including differences among payer sources, utilization, and payment mechanisms and what this means to hospice patients and their families, is very useful in the clinician's role. This includes understanding primary, secondary, and comorbid diagnoses; related supplies/medications/equipment/services; criteria for changes in levels of care; and the impact of a hospice election on the patient's Medicare benefit.

- Time-management skills to be able to prioritize and manage diverse and sometimes equally important tasks and responsibilities

  The best clinicians in hospice are very well organized and use their organizational skills in their daily routines. They create and keep detailed schedules, document at the patient's home (unless there are safety concerns), and generally seek to do things right the first time. Technological tools, such as scheduling systems and text/email, can assist these important aspects of communication and care.

- The practical wisdom of hospice care and practice

  Practical wisdom is information that comes with reading and practice. It may be called "the best way to do things." Much of this knowledge base comes from watching and learning from experienced hospice nurses. It includes such practical tips as always having two supplies with you (the Noah's Ark approach) because the time you don't will be the time you need that second catheter or another item. Other areas where experience helps include organizing paperwork, setting up your schedule, and tracking physician orders. Try to impart to others the information you needed when you began and have now.

## HOSPICE ORIENTATION: CONSIDERATIONS FOR SUCCESS

All new hospice team members need an appropriate orientation period. A high-quality orientation is important to being successful and feeling comfortable in the hospice team member role. No matter how understaffed the program may be, prospective team members should, when possible, try to define or address their orientation (including time span and content) before accepting the position. The following list addresses some of the information that an orientation should include. Obviously, if the clinician or manager has been in hospice for some time, it may not be appropriate or necessary to review all this information; however, it is important that all team members understand these hallmarks of hospice.

- The organization's orientation manual
- The Medicare CoPs for Hospice (or Home Health Care if the organization is a dually Medicare-certified program)
- The Medicare hospice or HHA manuals (the coverage of services sections) if the organization is a Medicare-certified hospice or HHA
- The hospice clinical and administrative policy and procedure manual(s)
- The schedule of hospice team meetings and staff support meetings
- An overview of the organization's clinical records and electronic health record/documentation system and required forms, including where, when, and how documentation is submitted
- Guidelines for home visits and what they entail, including verbal orders, the referral process, and scheduling
- The opportunity to "buddy" or precept with an experienced clinician
- Hospice coverage and documentation requirements, including confidentiality and the timeliness of physician orders
- Administrative details and processes (for example, payroll, on-call scheduling, and mileage reporting)
- Equipment and supply acquisitions (for example, nursing supplies and personal protective equipment [PPE])
- Performance improvement activities and processes and the clinician's role in identifying and reporting information (for example, infections, falls, missed visits, and adverse drug reactions)
- Benefits, employee handbook, mileage, on-call process and pay, lab pick-up schedules, and other miscellaneous information unique to the program

- Occupational Safety and Health Administration (OSHA) requirements, including (1) hepatitis B virus vaccination, (2) organizational policies and supplies for bloodborne pathogens and tuberculosis, (3) standard precaution supplies with appropriate barriers and related disposal of supplies, and (4) record-keeping activities
- Completion of a skills checklist or proficiency testing and ongoing educational plan
- Information related to compliance with laws and regulations (for example, home health aide supervision and timeliness for obtaining physician orders)
- Pain and symptom-management skills
- An orientation to the hospice's emergency preparedness program
- On-call strategies and skills
- The roles of the other team members of the hospice interdisciplinary group
- Training on the Medicare hospice regulations and state hospice licensure regulations

## HOSPICE ORIENTATION CONSIDERATIONS

Hospice orientation varies in scope, depth, and time span, depending on the organization and the new team member's experience. Remember that you are not alone in making the transition to a new area of care or practice and that orientation and education continue long after the formal orientation period. In fact, the best hospice team members and managers truly make learning a lifelong endeavor. There is always more to know!

Everyone knows how exciting and difficult it can be to leave what is known and familiar and move on to learn new skills in a foreign environment. The challenge is well worth the work. No clinician new to home healthcare or hospice should care for patients without an effective orientation. Orientation is perhaps the most important period in the role transformation to hospice, and the initial information presented may set the stage for future growth, professional development, and the clinician's satisfaction in the role and the organization. The orientation period is the time designated for honing clinical skills, taking the time to find answers, and developing new relationships with peers and managers. Perry Paxton said, "Excellence is in the details. Give attention to the details and excellence will come" (Paxton, n.d.). This is very true in hospice care. During orientation, the information is provided about documentation, detailed assessments, thoughtful data analysis, and the importance of clear communications. These kinds of details contribute to effective and quality hospice care. Perhaps most important, orientation is the time to be detail-oriented and acquire the knowledge that constitutes the "practical wisdom" of hospice.

## DEFINING THE HOSPICE ORIENTATION

Many important aspects of hospice care must be covered in the limited "official" orientation period. Overall behavioral outcomes or goals for the transitioning clinician include:

- Completing the orientation within the time allocated
- Identifying key staff members and customers (defined by the organization)
- Describing and explaining new patient assignment processes
- Demonstrating clinical competence in the home hospice setting
- Adhering to policies and procedures as observed/monitored
- Knowing where to go for questions or challenges related to practice and operations
- Other goals defined by the individual hospice organization

## COMPETENCY ASSESSMENT AND VALIDATION

Employees new to hospice can expect their new or existing employer to check their references and request completion of a self-assessment tool or checklist. These checklists identify specific skills or areas of knowledge and education, including areas where the clinician may need to review or be observed. They are also a way to validate competency, which is a hallmark of quality in hospice practice. The process of identifying educational and orientation needs is a way for the organization to ensure competency by hiring qualified team members.

Some organizations identify their own list of high-risk, low-volume skills and may have all nurses demonstrate competency in these skills. Examples include tracheotomy care and specialty assessments. A preceptor may accompany the new clinician in the field to observe certain skills and thereby ensure safe and effective patient care and standardization of care and care processes among team members and across the organization.

## ORGANIZATIONAL ORIENTATION TOPICS

The topics that may be addressed by the organization's orientation program cover a broad range of content. The information under these topics is prioritized in this section to emphasize the regulatory aspects interfacing with clinical patient care that must be understood to function safely in hospice. This section then lists topics and areas that should be addressed for quality, safety, practice, and accreditation reasons.

Although this looks like a voluminous amount of information, it all will make sense over the months to come. In fact, colleagues who have successfully made the transition are likely to say that "about 6 months into this, it all came together." This information is presented in a functional format to make sense to clinicians making this important transition. There are numerous policies in hospice, but those listed here, and their associated processes/outcomes, provide a practical overview of the hospice specialty. This list is by no means all-inclusive, but it identifies those areas with the most direct impact on hospice teams.

### Safety in Hospice

Personal safety is an appropriate concern in community-based practice. It is particularly important to team members entering unfamiliar geographical areas or at unusual hours. The clinician should review any protocols the hospice organization has related to staff safety and home visits. Organizational procedures such as communicating schedules may assist in staff safety. Some organizations have local law enforcement that provides training and education about home visiting and safety. The information shared is valuable to team members both as clinicians and as members of a community.

Personal safety starts with awareness of the surroundings. (See the "Personal Safety Tips" and "Car Safety Tips" sidebars for a list of safety tips.) Use those well-honed skills of observation and assessment wherever you are.

## PERSONAL SAFETY TIPS

- When going anywhere for the first time, get specific, detailed, and correct directions to the patient's home and have them validated by the patient or caregiver.

- If you are unsure of a neighborhood or have heard about problems, talk with your supervisor, who may contact the local police. The police know the communities and the problems best and can be very helpful in identifying problem areas and working with the care team on solutions.

- Organizations may have contracts with security staff. Your supervisor will know of such arrangements and the process for their use.

- Know the community. As you are driving, always be aware of your surroundings.

- You may want to call patients and families before leaving so they can be watching for you. Ask about parking as well.

- Lock the car doors and keep any valuables, such as purse, supplies, and any patient information, out of sight.

- Wear a seatbelt while driving.

- Try to park in well-lit areas and in front of the home or as close as possible. Lock the car and identify your route to the front door.

- Be cautious when boarding elevators.

*(continues)*

*(continued)*

- Have your needed supplies in an accessible area so you are not searching in the trunk for a needed supply.

- When making evening or night visits, let your family know where you are going and when you expect to return.

- When walking to your car, have your keys out, ready to unlock the car.

- Before getting back in the car, check the back seat and floor areas.

- Lock the car after re-entering, and proceed to a safe place.

- Trust your intuition. If you feel unsafe, call your supervisor or the police from a safe location.

- Speak with your supervisor about your organization's unique policies relating to home visit safety.

## CAR SAFETY TIPS

Car safety begins with knowledge of the strengths and weaknesses of your car. Successful and safe home visiting team members have good driving records and reliable cars that are usually fuel-efficient. A small car can be easier to park in congested areas, whereas a heavier car may perform better in bad weather.

- Keep a full tank. Try to never let the tank go below half-full.

- Carry water, a blanket, and a first aid kit. In cold weather, consider carrying a candle and a coffee can for careful use to provide heat if you become stranded.

- Keep all supplies secured so they do not become hazards in the event of quick braking or collisions.

- Lock all doors when entering or leaving your vehicle.

- If your organization gives you a sign that identifies you as a healthcare provider, use it according to organizational policies.

- Consider purchasing emergency roadside assistance through your insurance provider or AAA.

- Take good care of your vehicle providing all recommended maintenance. Winterize it if you live in areas that may reach freezing temperatures.

- Make sure that your spare tire is in good condition and inflated. Have the tools, knowledge, and ability to change a flat tire.

## Emergency Preparedness Program

The hospice organization should have an emergency preparedness plan in case the normal operations of the organization or office are disrupted. Examples of emergencies might include fire, severe weather, active shooter, power outages, and others unique to your area. Patient care should continue to the extent possible with patients prioritized based on their needs. Hospice team members should know their roles and activities in the process. Emergency command structure, communication plans, patient information with assigned priority codes, and drills should all be a part of the emergency preparedness and safety plan.

## Ethics in Hospice

It is important for hospice providers to institute ethical guidelines that will help assess accountability to the individuals and the communities they serve. An organization with clearly articulated ethical principles and a thorough commitment to those principles is better positioned to respond more effectively in times of crisis and change than one without such guidelines.

Increasing awareness of individual and organizational ethics can build a culture infused with trust and compliance with regulations. It also encourages a commitment to a sustained ethical environment that can be a direct force in heightening excellence and morale in any organization (NHPCO, 2016).

The National Hospice and Palliative Care Organization (NHPCO) has developed ethical principles in the hospice and palliative care community by outlining guiding principles for internal and external relations. These principles are available to hospice and palliative care providers to assist them in developing an organization built on trust and doing the right thing for patients, families, employees, volunteers, governing boards, referral sources, donors, and the general public (NHPCO, 2016).

- NHPCO Ethical Principles (https://www.nhpco.org/ethical-principles)
- Hospice team self-care

  Caring for people at the end of life is meaningful and fulfilling, but it can take a toll on the IDG. The hospice team experiences stress on a daily basis as they guide their patients and families through the end-of-life experience.

  The IDG provides valuable support to patients and families. It is important for them to process their feelings, particularly grief, so they do not become burned out. Common signs of burnout can include:

  - Irritability and impatience
  - Anxiety or depression
  - Poor sleep
  - Forgetfulness
  - Somatic symptoms, such as headaches and gastrointestinal distress
  - Reduction or increase in appetite and food intake
  - Increased illness
- Self-care methods for hospice professionals include:
  - Engage in rejuvenating activities such as a nature walk, time with a good friend, or a fitness activity.
  - Learn to set boundaries, and only say yes to what you have the energy to do.
  - Build a support team.

- Get more sleep. Take naps, if able.
- Listen to soothing music.
- Journal about your experiences.
- Vent about your feelings to someone who is willing to listen.
- If you have a spiritual practice, use it.
- Get a massage or another form of relaxation/pampering.
- Give yourself permission to be human (Weinstein, 2016).

# TRENDS IN HOSPICE CARE: STAYING APPRISED AND ENGAGED

The following areas are continuing challenges for the hospice industry.

## LENGTH OF STAY

Although more people are seeking end-of-life care, the number of short stays in hospice is increasing. A 2013 report from the NHPCO shows that more than one in three hospice patients (35.5%) died or were discharged within 7 days of admission last year. NHPCO is concerned about the rising percentage of patients spending 1 week or less in hospice because these patients and their family do not have the opportunity to experience the wide range of benefits during such a short time. A literature review completed by NHPCO shows that there are three major themes on why patients do not enter hospice earlier:

- **Hospice-eligible patient decision-making**—Patient and family readiness are factors as is the general acceptance of the end of life.

- **Racial and ethnic differences among hospice-eligible patients**—Underutilization of hospice among low-income, urban Hispanic/Latino, and African-American families may, in part, be due to cultural beliefs of familial provision of care to the dying.

- **Role of the physician**—Physicians tend to delay the discussion of hospice with patients about end of life. Additional physician barriers include a lack of knowledge of hospice admissions and election criteria, family dynamics, and insufficient hospice program marketing (NHPCO, 2013c).

## LIVE DISCHARGE

A patient may be discharged alive from hospice for several reasons. The Medicare hospice regulations allow a live discharge for the following reasons:

- The beneficiary decides to revoke the hospice benefit.
- The patient moves out of the hospice's service area or transfers to another hospice.
- The hospice determines that the patient is no longer terminally ill.
- The patient is discharged for cause (discussed earlier in this chapter).

The hospice must have a discharge planning process in place that considers the prospect of a patient's condition stabilizing or otherwise changing such that the patient cannot continue to be certified as terminally ill. The discharge planning process must include planning for any necessary family counseling, patient education, or other services before the patient is discharged because he or she is no longer terminally ill (CMS, 2005).

CMS is currently monitoring live discharge rates in hospice that have been increasing over the past decade. Live discharges are monitored and reported in the annual PEPPER report that is prepared and available to all Medicare-certified hospice providers. The Program for Evaluating Payment Patterns Electronic Report (PEPPER) is a contracted service provided for CMS that gives provider-specific Medicare data statistics for discharges/services vulnerable to improper payments (Program for Evaluating Payment Patterns Electronic Report, 2017).

## HOSPICE DATA

For benchmarking purposes, you can look up the National Hospice and Palliative Care Organization's (NHPCO) "Facts and Figures: Hospice Care in America" report, which provides a yearly review and overview of significant trends in the growth, delivery, and quality of hospice care across the country (NHPCO, 2015b).

## ADVANCE CARE PLANNING

An advance directive is a document by which a person makes his or her wishes known regarding healthcare in the event of being unable to make those decisions. There are two main types of advance directive: the Living Will and the Durable Power of Attorney for Health Care. Advance care planning is about discussing, deciding, and documenting an individual's wishes and preferences about healthcare interventions if he or she is unable to make those decisions or speak for themselves. Several written documents are available to express care wishes and/or appoint a surrogate decision-maker. It is important to ensure that the designated surrogate knows and understands the individual's care preferences and agrees to carry them out. Development of an advance care plan can help lessen unnecessary suffering, improve quality of life, and provide better understanding of the decision-making challenges facing the individual and the caregivers. An advance care plan can be developed and used at any age and should be updated as an individual's circumstances change (Centers for Disease Control and Prevention, n.d.).

Advance care planning begins with a conversation between an individual and the physician and involves discussion of disease trajectory and related conditions. The goal of advance care planning is to try to proactively make decisions when an individual is well and not in active disease crises. Advance care planning is especially important if a patient does not want aggressive treatment and hospice providers honor an individual's plan or provide the individual with the information to form a plan if there is not one already (Centers for Disease Control and Prevention, n.d.).

Laws vary from state to state, so it is important to be familiar with the tools used in your area. Documents such as the Physician Orders for Life Sustaining Treatment (POLST) and others may guide your practice area.

# SUMMARY

Hospice is a type of palliative care that provides quality, compassionate care for people facing a serious life-limiting illness or injury per their wishes or advance care plan. Trends that are noted in hospice care over the past decade are increasing short length of stay and live discharge even though more people are choosing hospice care at end of life. Regulations are in place at the federal and state levels for hospice providers, and some providers seek additional accreditation. Medicare has also implemented quality reporting requirements and caregiver satisfactions surveys for hospice providers and has implemented public reporting to align them with other providers under the Medicare umbrella.

Hospice is a growing area that combines the best of skillful, compassionate care and respect for patient and family choices at the end of life while working within the confines of federal and state regulatory frameworks.

## References

Centers for Disease Control and Prevention. (n.d.). Advance care planning: Ensuring your wishes are known and honored if you are unable to speak for yourself. Retrieved from https://www.cdc.gov/aging/pdf/advanced-care-planning-critical-issue-brief.pdf

Centers for Medicare and Medicaid Services. (1983). Medicare program; hospice care. Retrieved from https://www.cms.gov/Medicare/Medicare-Fee-for-Service-Payment/Hospice/Downloads/1983-Final-Rule.pdf

Centers for Medicare and Medicaid Services. (2005). Medicare program; hospice care amendments. Retrieved from https://www.cms.gov/Regulations-and-Guidance/Regulations-and-Policies/QuarterlyProviderUpdates/Downloads/cms1022f.pdf

Centers for Medicare and Medicaid Services. (2008). Medicare and Medicaid programs: Hospice conditions of participation. Retrieved from https://www.gpo.gov/fdsys/pkg/FR-2008-06-05/pdf/08-1305.pdf

Centers for Medicare and Medicaid Services. (2013). Medicare program; FY 2014 hospice wage index and payment rate update; hospice quality reporting requirements; and updates on payment reform; final rule. Retrieved from https://www.gpo.gov/fdsys/pkg/FR-2013-08-07/pdf/2013-18838.pdf

Centers for Medicare and Medicaid Services. (2015a). Medicare program; FY 2016 hospice wage index and payment rate update and hospice quality reporting requirements; final rule. Retrieved from https://www.gpo.gov/fdsys/pkg/FR-2015-08-06/pdf/2015-19033.pdf

Centers for Medicare and Medicaid Services. (2015b). Medicare Benefit Policy Manual, Chapter 9 - Coverage of Hospice Services under Hospital Insurance. Retrieved from https://www.cms.gov/Regulations-and-Guidance/Guidance/Manuals/Downloads/bp102c09.pdf

Centers for Medicare and Medicaid Services. (2016). Medicare program; FY 2017 hospice wage index and payment rate update and hospice quality reporting requirements; final rule. Retrieved from https://s3.amazonaws.com/public-inspection.federalregister.gov/2016-18221.pdf

Connor, S. R. (2008). Development of hospice and palliative care in the United States. *OMEGA-Journal of Death and Dying, 56*(1), 89–99.

Davis, F. A. (1988). Medicare hospice benefit: Early program experiences. *Health Care Financing Review, 9*(4), 99–111.

Goebel, J. R., Doering, L. V., Lorenz, K. A., Maliski, S. L., Nyamathi, A. M., & Evangelista, L. S. (2009). Caring for special populations: Total pain theory in advanced heart failure: Applications to research and practice. *Nursing Forum, 44*(3), 175–185. doi:10.1111/j.1744-6198.2009.00140.x

Hospice & Palliative Credentialing Center. (2014). Why certification: Claiming and validating our expertise. Retrieved from http://advancingexpertcare.org/why-certification/

Institute of Medicine. (2014). Dying in America: Improving quality and honoring individual preferences near the end of life. Retrieved from http://iom.nationalacademies.org/Reports/2014/Dying-In-America-Improving-Quality-and-Honoring-Individual-Preferences-Near-the-End-of-Life.aspx

Medicare Payment Advisory Commission. (2015, March). Report to the Congress: Medicare payment policy: Hospice. Retrieved from http://www.medpac.gov/docs/default-source/reports/chapter-12-hospice-services-march-2015-report-.pdf?sfvrsn=0

Medicare Payment Advisory Commission. (2016, March). Report to the Congress: Medicare payment policy: Hospice. Retrieved from http://www.medpac.gov/docs/default-source/reports/chapter-11-hospice-services-march-2016-report-.pdf?sfvrsn=0

National Hospice and Palliative Care Organization. (2011). *Hospice care: Physician's guide.* Alexandria, VA: NHPCO.

National Hospice and Palliative Care Organization. (2013a). Preamble to NHPCO standards of practice. Retrieved from http://www.nhpco.org/ethical-and-position-statements/preamble-and-philosophy

National Hospice and Palliative Care Organization. (2013b). Care continuum. Retrieved from http://www.nhpco.org/care-continuum

National Hospice and Palliative Care Organization. (2013c, November). Short length of stay literature review. Retrieved from http://www.hospiceactionnetwork.org/linked_documents/HAN_in_action/HAN_events/symposium/Short_LOS_Lit_Review.pdf

National Hospice and Palliative Care Organization. (2015a). Hospice care. Retrieved from http://www.nhpco.org/about/hospice-care

National Hospice and Palliative Care Organization. (2015b). NHPCO's facts and figures hospice care in America: 2015 edition. Retrieved from http://www.nhpco.org/sites/default/files/public/Statistics_Research/2016_Facts_Figures.pdf

National Hospice and Palliative Care Organization. (2016). Guide to organizational ethics in hospice care. Retrieved from https://www.nhpco.org/files/guide-organizational-ethics-hospice-care

Paxton, P. (n.d.). Retrieved from http://www.quotationreference.com/
quotefinder.php?byax=1&strt=1&subj=Perry+Paxton

Program for Evaluating Payment Patterns Electronic Report. (2017). PEPPER resources.
Retrieved from https://pepperresources.org/

Rome, R. B., Luminais, H. H., Bourgeois, D. A., & Blais, C. M. (2011). The role of palliative
care at the end of life. *The Ochsner Journal, 11*(4), 348–352.

Stanford School of Medicine. (2016). Where do Americans die? Retrieved from
https://palliative.stanford.edu/home-hospice-home-care-of-the-dying-patient/
where-do-americans-die/

Weinstein, E. (2016). Caregiver burnout: The importance of self care. *Psych Central.*
Retrieved from https://psychcentral.com/lib/caregiver-burnout-the-importance-
of-self-care/

# Documentation: An Important Driver for Care and Coverage

Part 2 seeks to assist both new and experienced hospice nurses and other team members in meeting various requirements and documenting the specific information required by any payer; "paint a picture" of the patient's/family's conditions, concerns, care and responses to care, and interventions; and overall, to accurately chronicle the patient's individualized hospice care.

## HOSPICE DOCUMENTATION: WHY IS THE CLINICAL RECORD SO IMPORTANT?

The hospice clinical record is a legal document and is the only one that chronicles a patient's stay from admission and start of hospice care through to death or discharge. If the agency has computerized clinical records, the data might be entered at the point of care with the patient and family. It is strongly recommended that the documentation be completed as soon as possible and at the time the care is provided, when possible, to ensure accuracy of the information. The care and practice of hospice team members are described every day to surveyors, peers, and managers in the hospice clinical record. Visit records, notes, and other information that appears in the record reflect the standard of hospice care as well as the unique care provided to a specific patient and family.

Hospice team members must be able to integrate the knowledge of regulatory criteria, care coordination, and practice into effective documentation that supports coverage while demonstrating quality and value to any reviewer. Third-party payers, such as the Medicare Administrative Contractors (MACs), make numerous quality and reimbursement decisions based on the care the patient received as evidenced in the hospice clinical record. Other reviewers might include accreditation bodies, state licensure surveyors, federal auditors, consultants, and others. For these reasons, hospice team members must have an effective understanding of the hospice regulatory environment and the expectations about the standards of effective hospice documentation. When in doubt, ask your supervisor about the hospice's policies and requirements related to documentation.

The following sections discuss factors that contribute to hospice documentation.

## INCREASED SCRUTINY OF HOSPICE SERVICES

A clinician's documentation plays a critical role in today's hospice environment. Documentation of hospice care must be complete, accurate, detailed, and consistent enough to tell the patient's and family's story. There is huge federal and state focus on healthcare fraud and abuse as an outcome of the 2010 Affordable Care Act (ACA). This increases the probability of a hospice receiving this type of audit. These audits would be separate from a recertification or relicensure survey. Targeted audits from commercial insurance companies or payers have also risen in the past decade. The quality and comprehensiveness of documentation determines the outcome of any audit, such as those for survey and certification and licensure. Financial payback is on the line, and because of this, hospices need to educate clinicians about hospice-specific documentation regulatory requirements, identify and set documentation standards, and hold clinicians accountable for care and the related documentation.

Because Medicare is the largest payer for hospice services in the United States, its interest in ensuring that fraud and abuse in the Medicare system is identified and limited is very high. These "federal" or government dollars belong to everyone collectively as tax payers. All have a vested interest in these limited dollars being spent in the most effective way.

Hospice utilization has been under analysis since 2013, and the Center for Medicare and Medicaid Services (CMS) is concerned about the cost of services provided to Medicare beneficiaries, including those provided outside of the hospice benefit. This includes Medicare Parts A, B, and D. As hospice utilization rises and the number of providers increases, continued focus from CMS and other regulatory and fiduciary entities will continue. The Office of the Inspector General (OIG) updates its annual plan in the fall for the following year. Visit https://oig.hhs.gov/ for information related to definitions and examples of fraud or other activities under scrutiny related to hospice. This might include metrics such as hospice utilization in assisted living facilities, general patient use and billing, hospice in a nursing facility setting, and more. In this environment of scrutiny, it is more important than ever for patient documentation to clearly reflect the patient's hospice status and the specific nursing and other medically necessary care provided because the ability to receive and retain payment depends on this clarity, quality, and value.

## THE EMPHASIS ON QUALITY ASSESSMENT AND PERFORMANCE IMPROVEMENT (QAPI)

When the CMS revised the Conditions of Participation (CoPs) in 2008, the focus of the regulations was on the care delivered to patients and their families by the hospice team and the outcome(s) of that care. The CoPs are based on four core requirements. These are:

- Patient rights
- Comprehensive assessment
- Patient care planning
- Coordination by a hospice interdisciplinary group (IDG)

The four core requirements are guided by the hospice's QAPI program, where quality management is the key to improved patient care performance. The intent of the regulation is to ensure that a hospice provides patient care that meets essential health and quality standards, while ensuring that it monitors and improves its own hospice performance organization-wide. The CoPs focus on the core requirements and are deemed necessary by CMS to attain positive patient outcomes and to meet the increasing challenges associated with the hospice care environment. The regulatory intent is based on the following principles:

- Emphasis on patient/family experiences across the hospice continuum of care and on activities that center on patient assessment, care planning, service delivery, quality assessment, and performance improvement

- Incorporate and implement an outcome-oriented quality assessment and performance improvement program

- Use performance measurement systems to evaluate and improve care (CMS, 2008)

## THE EMPHASIS ON STANDARDIZATION OF CARE, POLICIES AND PROCEDURES, AND PROCESSES

Patients are entitled to a certain level or standard of care. Operationally, this means that regardless of which clinician is assigned and providing care, the patient receives generally the same level of care and the same interventions in the same order as designated by the organization and its managers. This helps ensure standardization of care and related processes across the organization. This also helps ensure the same "brand" and level of quality hospice care is provided in a community by all team members. In fact, the use of a text, such as this, by all clinicians at a given hospice organization contributes to such standardization of patient care. Other examples would be all team members using the same medication resources, clinical policy and procedure manuals, and more. Such processes put everyone "on the same page" from a quality and clinical perspective.

## RECOGNITION AND EMPOWERMENT OF THE NURSING PROFESSION AND THE NURSING SHORTAGE

The landmark Institute of Medicine (IOM) report "The Future of Nursing: Leading Change, Advancing Health" heralded a new vision for

**TABLE 2.1** Benefits and Challenges of an EHR

| Benefits | Challenges |
| --- | --- |
| Promotes legible, complete documentation and accurate, streamlined translation to coding and billing | Not enough detail (appears standardized) |
| | Check boxes or radio controls that reduce patient specificity |
| Provides accurate, up-to-date, and complete information about patients at the point of care | Inconsistent between disciplines (appears multidisciplinary versus interdisciplinary) |
| Provides a mechanism for secure sharing of electronic information with patients and other clinicians | Interoperability and data exchange (systems cannot communicate with each other) |
| Saves space related to a digital records environment | Expense for system purchase and implementation |
| Enables quick access to patient records for more coordinated, efficient care provision | Safety and liability (HIPAA security requirements) |
| Helps providers improve staff productivity and enables improved efficiency | Requires increased training of staff |
| Allows easier collection and trending of data | Data entry is not always intuitive and may require work-arounds |

Reference: HealthIT.gov (2014), https://www.healthit.gov/providers-professionals/faqs/what-are-advantages-electronic-health-records

## IMPORTANCE OF THE HOSPICE PATIENT RECORD

The importance of documentation in the clinical record relates to the fact that this record has the following characteristics:

- It is the formal written record of reference of care interventions, coordination of care, and communication among members of the hospice care team and external sources
- It is the text that supports justification for insurance reimbursement

- It is the evidence on which patient care decisions were based
- It is the only legal record
- It is the primary foundation for the evaluation of the care provided
- It is the basis for staff education or quality assessment and performance improvement (QAPI) purposes
- It is the objective source for an organization's licensing, where applicable, certification and accreditation, state survey, or other reviews or audits

Simply stated, the documentation is the point at which a theory or idea is tested from a quality, medical necessity, coverage standpoint, and evidences the many other nuances of providing the best hospice care.

CMS manages the Medicare program and instructs state survey agencies on the administration of the Medicare Hospice Benefit and MACs on the reimbursement for Medicare hospice services. Of course, these instructions have huge implications for hospice team members who provide care to patients covered under the Medicare Hospice Benefit. These intermediaries contract with the CMS to process and make payment determinations on hospice and homecare claims from across the country. The payers can pay only for hospice care under Medicare provisions that are covered by law. The payers look to the hospice clinical documentation in the medical record to determine whether they support the tenets and rules of covered appropriate hospice care. For hospice to be covered under Medicare, services must meet the following requirements.

- They must be reasonable and necessary for the palliation and management of the terminal illness as well as related conditions.
- The individual must elect hospice care in accordance with §418.24.
- A plan of care must be established and periodically reviewed by the attending physician, the medical director, and the interdisciplinary group of the hospice program as set forth in §418.56. That plan of care must be established before hospice care is provided.
- The services provided must be consistent with the plan of care.
- A certification that the individual is terminally ill must be completed as set forth in §418.22.

- A hospice provider's inability to evidence compliance with conditions of coverage can be used as a basis for payment denial by the provider's MAC. This requirement is specifically documented in Chapter 3 of the Medicare Program Integrity (the "IOM Manual"). (http://www.cms.gov/Regulations-and-Guidance/Guidance/Manuals/downloads/pim83c03.pdf)

Recent hospice industry data trends identified by CMS and individual provider data and investigation have increased scrutiny of hospice by the federal government. Because of this heightened review, it's more important than ever that hospices and hospice team members know the rules, effectively document patient care, and manage their hospice clinical records. All state, federal government, and Medicare reviewers hold Medicare-participating hospice organizations accountable for compliance with the Medicare hospice regulations.

# DOCUMENTATION: THE KEY TO CARE, COVERAGE, COMPLIANCE, AND QUALITY

Documentation is critical to the positive outcome of any review process. Paint a picture with your documentation from the onset of care through the continuation of hospice services through to the patient's discharge or death. Distinguish clearly in your documentation between the chronic phases of a disease, especially if it is a long and slow decline. Document patient periods of exacerbation, stabilization, and deterioration. Document the way treatments and medications play a palliative role in the patient's plan of care and actual management of symptoms. Remember, all team member notes are usually assessed during a review, and all documentation should paint a clear picture of the patient and the patient's family to meet the criteria for the Medicare Hospice Benefit. Even if a patient experiences a period of disease plateau or stabilization, the patient may still be terminally ill and eligible for hospice care. Documentation should not include generalizations such as the terms "no change" or "as tolerated" because these are vague terms and do not assist in painting a picture of a terminally ill individual. The reviewer would not understand and "see" what is truly happening with your hospice patient.

## HOSPICE DOCUMENTATION: THE FUNDAMENTALS

Medicare, like any medical insurance program, has both covered services and exclusions. For payers, documentation may be the only trail of the care provided and the patient's response to that care. As explained in Part 1, it is imperative that clinicians and managers understand the Medicare Hospice Benefit. The objective information that paints the picture of an appropriate patient for the Medicare hospice program is supported by a clinician's documentation in the patient's record. This may include the hospice admission history and physical findings: the detailed assessment, the hospice election form with designated effective dates, the certifications of the terminal illness with clinical facts, and interdisciplinary group notes. This data can help support the appropriateness of the admission and continuing hospice service. Other notes would include interdisciplinary visit notes, the patient's prognosis, and many other kinds of findings describing the patient condition, the family's response to care, the patient's response to interventions, and numerous other indicators of quality hospice care. Other important information would be patient diagnoses; comorbidities that impact the prognoses; the history and progression of the patient's illness, including the physical findings and baseline such as weight/weight changes, heart rhythms, rales, edema sites and amounts; and other objective measures.

## DOCUMENTATION TIPS FOR PAPER-BASED DOCUMENTATION

Some documentation is a blend of EMR and paper-based documentation. For that reason, the following are some documentation tips:

- Write legibly or print neatly; the record must be legible and readable. Do not let people guess what you said or what they thought you said. What you have to say is incredibly important. Don't diminish the value of your contribution to this patient's care by writing illegibly. Subsequent care decisions are made on this information.

- Use permanent ink; sometimes an organization requires a specific color such as black or blue as part of policy.

- For every entry, identify the time and date, sign the entry, and include your name and credentials legibly.

- Use ink that does not smear and remains legible even if the document gets wet.

- Describe the specific care or interventions provided; mark appropriate boxes on flowsheets or other documentation tools and the patient's response to the care and interventions provided.

- Document in chronological order with no skipped areas.

- Try to document or enter data at the patient's home if it is safe; if this is not possible, document as soon as possible after the care interventions are provided.

- Be factual and specific.

- Use patient, family, or caregiver quotes to support the patient and family status.

- Use the patient's name, such as Mr. Smith.

- Document patient complaints and the resolution; remember to discuss any complaints with your manager, who may also document this in the complaint log and note the resolution or follow-up actions taken to be able to identify any trends.

- Make sure the patient's name is listed correctly on the visit record, for daily notes or other forms, and matches the information in the billing system.

- Be accurate, complete, and thorough.

- Write what you document in full, avoiding potentially confusing abbreviations.

- Chart only the care you provided.

- Promptly document any change in the patient's condition and the actions taken based on this change. It might be necessary to report a change in condition to the physician if it necessitates a change and update to the plan of care.

- Document the patient's, family's, or caregiver's response to teaching or any other care intervention.

- Review your organization's policy related to documentation corrections such as drawing a line through the erroneous entry or other policies.
- Try to avoid the following:
  - Relying on memory; this affects the accuracy of the documentation
  - Using correction fluid or erasing any entries
  - Crossing out words beyond recognition
  - Making assumptions or drawing conclusions and blaming
  - Documenting a judgment statement, such as "house is filthy" or "patient is angry"
  - Leaving blank spaces between entries and your signature
  - Waiting too long to record entries about care and interventions and the patient's/family's response to care and interventions
  - Leaving gaps in the documentation; intervals in documentation contribute to an inconsistent picture of the patient/family
  - Using abbreviations except where they are clear and appear on the organization's list of approved acceptable abbreviations
- When in doubt, check or ask about your organization's policies related to documentation.

## DOCUMENTATION TIPS FOR ELECTRONIC HEALTH RECORDS

Electronic health records bring different challenges and attributes to documentation. The following are some tips for electronic documentation.

- Increase detail in electronic documentation.
  - Expand on point-and-click selections in a note.
  - Record observations about selections in available drop-down menus. (For example, state the number of feet a patient can ambulate.)
  - Where needed, individualize the information about the patient. (For example, after check boxes are completed, add entries that describe the patient.)

- Individualize care that describes a unique picture of the patient and family.

  - Document subjective comments from the patient and family to support continued eligibility. (For example, "I sat outside last week, but this week I just don't have the energy to go out" and "My clothes are so loose now that my sister went and bought me new shirts.")

  - Do not use the cut and paste option if it is available.

  - Ensure that all IDG members review each other's documentation to promote consistency and congruency.

  - Never communicate secure logins or passwords to unauthorized persons.

  - Only document about a patient in a device that is protected by the organization's program and security.

  - Only have one patient chart open at a time to avoid incorrect entries.

## DOCUMENTATION QUALITY AND VALUE CONSIDERATIONS

Whether systems-based, paper records, or a blend of both, the quality of a provider's documentation is just as important as the quality of care he/she provides to the patient and family. Effective documentation is objective, concise, authentic, timely, comprehensive but pertinent, and consistent. Such documentation tells the patient's and family's unique story. Quality documentation includes:

- Observations and descriptions of the patient's condition

  - Pain and symptom assessments and management/interventions

  - Changes or findings to use in care planning and communication with other IDG members

- Observations and descriptions of family or caregiver status

- Observations about the patient's environment of care and how that environment supports the care or acts as an impediment to the plan of care

- A comprehensive description of care/services, interventions, the patient/family response to the care/interventions, and evaluations of the care provided
- Patient/family response to specific interventions and care
- All communication with the physician and other IDG team members
- Needed detail to paint the picture of the patient's condition
- Patient appearance and description of pain, and other distress/symptoms/findings; this is especially true when there are differences and changes

Use prognostic tools accurately. Use the right tool for the right diagnosis or problem and in the right way.

Ensure that information included in summaries, narratives, and prognostic worksheets is supported by visit or other encounter (continuous care or other care) documentation.

# DOCUMENTATION STRATEGIES

A clinician can use several strategies to achieve higher quality documentation. One fundamental strategy is that quality documentation contains enough detail to be defensible to surveys and audits. This means it makes sense and truly paints a picture of the hospice patient and family and their care and trajectory/course of care across time. Teaching hospice staff to proactively complete effective documentation with quality helps organizations with concerns, such as if clinical records are reviewed by federal or state entities.

## FOCUSED DOCUMENTATION

Focused documentation is beneficial because it focuses on the patient's/family's status and needs from a specific and individualized viewpoint. This method requires the use of objective data and findings to support/evidence the patient's status at the time of the assessment and throughout care. This method of documentation is not restricted to nurses and can be employed by all IDG members.

The following examples depict a more focused documentation style:

- Document limits to activities of daily living for a patient with end-stage heart disease.
    - The patient can only tolerate sitting upright in a chair 2 hours per day per his caregiver.
- Describe the extent of oxygen for a patient with COPD and shortness of breath.
    - The patient experiences shortness of breath when walking more than 25 steps, even when using oxygen.

State facts with objective information and data reference if possible:

- Clothing no longer fits due to 10-pound weight loss.
- Sleeping occurs 12 hours per day.
- The patient states that pain increases from a 3 to a 6 when performing activities of daily living.
- The patient needs maximum assistance from two family members to be turned or repositioned due to frailty and patient distress when moved.

## COMPARATIVE DOCUMENTATION

The premise of a comparative documentation approach is focusing on one component at different points in time. The clinician compares and contrasts the patient's present condition to his/her prior condition. This comparison focuses on the patient's individualized trajectory of decline and presents specific information, not generalizations. Here are examples of comparative documentation:

- One week ago, Mr. Smith was eating one-half to three-quarters of two meals per day. This week he is eating one-quarter of one meal each day.
- Mr. Smith was able to sit up and watch TV last week; this week he reported "being too tired to even get up and sit in my TV chair" (CGS, 2013a, b).

## INCONSISTENT AND INSUFFICIENT DOCUMENTATION CONSIDERATIONS

There is an assumption made in this book that clinicians and other hospice team members have been provided a foundational level of orientation about hospice and hospice care. This includes coverage, documentation of hospice care and related requirements, care coordination required by the IDG, effective case management, pain and symptom management, use of objective tools available, how to make home visits, effective assessments, and numerous other hallmarks of quality hospice and its provision. This is required because providers need to ensure that documentation is consistent and sufficient among all the IDG members. Inconsistent and insufficient documentation does not adequately paint a picture of the patient and family, and it causes the documentation to appear inaccurate, uncoordinated, and irreconcilable to an objective reviewer. Simply put, it does not make sense and may be illegible and otherwise not meet standards for effective documentation that supports medically necessary hospice care.

The foundation of the hospice interdisciplinary group is that they work together toward a common goal through coordination with each other. This should be captured and reflected in the clinical notes. Any inconsistent or insufficient documentation should be scrutinized, discussed, and clarified/rectified through IDG coordination. Documentation that is not consistent or complete lacks sufficient detail to effectively support hospice eligibility and the terminal prognosis. A peer review or other process may assist in improving documentation. Simply put, poor documentation places an organization at risk. If a team member reads a note and cannot understand it or it raises more questions than it answers, there is a problem.

- Inconsistent documentation example—The nurse documents that a patient is nonambulatory on her visit, and the spiritual care professional documents that he walked with the patient in the hall 2 days later. Could this be possible? Possibly, but it appears to be inconsistent on the surface without additional detail. Perhaps the patient was not ambulatory for the nurse that day but was ambulatory

2 days later, or the spiritual care professional walked while pushing the patient in a wheelchair. Effective detail and care coordination is everything!

- Insufficient documentation example—This includes phrases like "slow, progressive decline," "appears to be losing weight," and "no change." The nurse documents that the patient is losing weight. That could mean any of the following:
  - The patient is eating less than before.
  - The patient is not eating at all.
  - The patient has lost 2 pounds.
  - The patient has lost 20 pounds or anywhere in between.
- Specify: use metrics and measurements—All this is to describe the detailed picture and tell the individual hospice patient and family's unique story!

## ACCURATE AND OBJECTIVE DOCUMENTATION

The clinical record is the specific and sole legal representation of the hospice care that the IDG provides to the patient and the family. Because of this, it must be an accurate, objective and detailed, individualized record of that care. Quality and accurate documentation records observations and subjective comments from the patient and family without conclusions or judgments. Again, inaccurate documentation does not adequately paint a picture of the patient and family, and it causes the documentation to appear inaccurate, uncoordinated, and irreconcilable to an objective reviewer. Here is an example of inaccurate hospice documentation:

- Excerpt from a spiritual care professional note: "Patient is sitting up in chair today and made eye contact with me for the whole visit. Patient listened to and smiled at prayers and hymns during visit, which made her happy."
- The reality: "This patient has advanced Alzheimer's disease and was propped up in a Geri chair with two pillows and a tray to keep her upright. She consistently displays a forward vacant stare no matter

what is in her line of vision and smiles no matter what is happening around her."

- The spiritual care professional's note was not detailed enough to be accurate about this specific patient. This patient could only sit in a chair because it was a specialty chair that kept her secure. She also needed the assistance of two pillows to keep her sitting upright. Also, the spiritual care professional drew conclusions by documenting that reciting prayers and singing hymns made this patient "happy."

# HOSPICE DOCUMENTATION RESOURCES

One key to effectively documenting or describing a patient at the end of life is to use and document data from objective symptom assessment scales and other clinical resources. Incorporating data outcomes and objective findings from these resources or tools evidences the patient's status, care needs, and decline. Any symptom management scale must be used consistently and accurately by clinical staff to ensure quality measurements and then support effective documentation.

## LOCAL COVERAGE DETERMINATIONS

A hospice provider's Medicare Administrative Contractor or MAC looks for the use or the reference of local coverage determinations (LCDs) in documentation during medical review of a hospice clinical record. The LCDs are specific guidelines, developed by the MAC, and not regulations per se. However, it is to a hospice's advantage to require staff to be knowledgeable about them and to incorporate them into their practice, care, and patient documentation. The LCDs include clinical criteria for various noncancer diagnoses, but hospice providers should not be so strict with their application that they bar eligible patients from receiving appropriate and medically necessary hospice care because the patient does not meet all the requirements of an LCD or there is not an LCD for the patient's unique disease process. Of course, when the LCDs are applied, patients who meet the criteria for an LCD are expected to have a 6-month or less prognosis if the terminal illness runs its normal course.

In addition, there may be patients who have a life expectancy of 6 months or less but do not meet any LCD guideline. Eligibility validation for these patients may be approved if the specific documentation of clinical factors evidences/supports a less than 6-month life expectancy. It is important to keep in mind that the noncancer LCDs are not the only diagnoses that can—or should be—used to determine whether a patient is eligible for hospice care. (Resource: Local Coverage Determinations [LCDs] by State Index.)

## SYMPTOM AND FUNCTIONALITY MEASUREMENT SCALES

It is also critical to apply and document patient outcomes of applicable symptom and functionality measurement scales. These data and outcomes paint a better picture of the patient's individualized care, status, and decline. Common scales used in symptom assessment include:

- Pain assessment—0–10 scale, Wong Face scale, and others
- New York Heart Association (NYHA) Functional Classification— It places patients in one of four categories based on how much they are limited during physical activity.
- Edmonton Symptom Assessment System (ESAS) Revised—This replaces the ESAS (2). The ESAS-r is freely available for use, with appropriate acknowledgment of its source.
- Modified Borg Scale for Perceived Dyspnea (shortness of breath)
- MMRC—Modified Medical Research Council Dyspnea Scale
- PPS—Palliative Performance Scale
- KPS—Karnofsky Performance Scale
- FAST—Functional Assessment Staging for Dementia
- MRI(S) —Mortality Risk Index (Score)
- ADEPT—Advanced Dementia Prognostic Tool
- Edmonton Frail Scale—https://www.nscphealth.co.uk/edmontonscale-pdf
- Others as hospices stay up to date on tools and resources

## SUPPORTING ELIGIBILITY AND TERMINAL PROGNOSIS

Documentation describes the picture of the patient. Often, the longer the patient's length of stay, the harder it becomes to evidence eligibility and decline in status. Patients with end-stage chronic illnesses can evidence slow general decline, so it is important to show a trajectory of that decline to support the terminal prognosis throughout the hospice election. Evidence of that decline could include:

- Weight change
- Diagnostic lab results (as ordered by physician)
- Changes in pain (type, location, frequency)
- Changes in responsiveness
- Changes in skin condition (turgor, bruising, edema, and so on)
- Changes in the level of dependence for ADLs
- Changes in anthropomorphic measurements (abdominal girth, upper arm measurements)
- Changes in vital signs (respiratory rate, blood pressure, pulse)
- Changes in strength
- Changes in lucidity
- Changes in intake/output
- Falls (patients in a weakened state or who are taking controlled drugs for symptom management are at a higher risk for falls and injury)
- Increasing emergent care visits or hospitalizations

## DECLINE, TERMINAL PLATEAUS, AND CHRONIC STATUS CONSIDERATIONS

As lengths of stay increase, the documentation of continued eligibility is critical and can sometimes become more difficult to document. Payers look specifically for evidence of appropriate and projected hospice patient decline. Questions reviewers or auditors may ask include (and you should look at this objectively):

- Is this patient terminal or chronic?
- Why is this patient still on hospice care?
- What clinical and other factors support that this unique patient is at end of life?
- Does documentation evidence a terminal prognosis and continued hospice eligibility?

The hospice LCDs include decline variables for a noncancer diagnosis and changes in clinical variables that apply to patients whose decline is not considered to be reversible. No minimum number of variables must be met for a patient to be eligible for hospice (CGS, 2013a).

The LCDs do include acknowledgment that patients in the terminal stage of an illness may display periods of stabilization and improve while receiving hospice care, yet have a reasonable expectation of continued decline for a life expectancy of less than 6 months, thus remaining eligible for hospice care. However, "if a patient improves or stabilizes sufficiently over time such that he/she no longer has a prognosis of six months or less from the most recent recertification evaluation or definitive interim evaluation, that patient should be considered for discharge from the Medicare Hospice Benefit" (NHPCO, 2010, p. 33).

It is critical that the hospice IDG documentation distinguish the patient experiencing "improvement" to chronic status from a period of stabilization yet clearly support, through data and documentation, that the patient is still terminal. This determination should be made patient by patient and with the hospice physician's decision in collaboration with the attending physician and IDG members. Discerning whether a plateau in decline is temporary or the disease has become chronic versus terminal is a hospice physician decision, but documenting evidence to support that decision is the responsibility of the entire IDG. This determination can be difficult, and the decision to discharge a patient because he or she no longer meets hospice eligibility is one made over time rather than in a moment.

Hospice providers should consider looking at the patient's status differently or with "new eyes" (objectively) to determine whether there is continuing patient decline. For example, a patient with congestive heart failure (CHF) who is on 2L of continuous oxygen lives in her bedroom and weighs 85 lbs. Her meals are brought to her, and she can only ambulate from her bed to a chair or commode chair. She experiences no shortness of breath, dizziness, or pain. She had no weight loss and no change in her appetite in the past 60 days. If the documentation states that she had no shortness of breath, dizziness, pain, weight loss, or change in appetite, visit after visit, it could be assumed that this patient is in a chronic state of illness rather than a terminal state of illness. But if the hospice team looks at this patient differently and documents differently, it would clearly evidence that the patient is hospice-eligible. Documenting that the patient has limited her living space and activity to an 8×8 space to control her symptoms speaks volumes, and it is these nuances that must be clearly communicated and carefully documented. One would not expect this patient to be routinely short of breath because her activity is minimal and has become so limited on purpose. In fact, she had no weight loss in the past 60 days because she had so little weight to lose.

Documenting interventions that control symptoms may seem obvious, but it can help support coverage and differentiate a chronic status from a terminal one. For example, documenting that the patient has no skin integrity problems because the caregiver is performing exceptional skin care helps support why this patient has no skin breakdown. Document what you are doing and what the family or others are doing that keeps the patient's symptoms effectively controlled. Some examples are:

- Patient has not been hospitalized because...
- Patient has no shortness of breath because...
- Patient does not have wounds, skin problems, or pressure injury because...

In other words, give yourself credit for skillful care to hospice patients and families that prevents problems.

Documenting specific interventions and care with rationales and out-comes provides the detail needed to evidence continued hospice eligibil-ity. This use of critical thinking/clinical reasoning is key to the provision of the best hospice care for patients and families.

## SUMMARY

Hospice team members play important roles in supporting coverage of hospice through effective and quality documentation. Overall, hospice documentation should reflect that the patient clearly has an illness of a terminal nature with a limited life expectancy of 6 months or less. The hospice documentation should emphasize the patient's prognosis what-ever the diagnosis; this is the reason for skillful hospice care and services. Hospice team members practicing in the community must be customer service-oriented, flexible, strong clinically, and able to document effec-tively to clearly paint a picture of the unique patient and family receiv-ing hospice care and services. Additional reviews and the emphasis on the collection of data quantifying the impact of care will only increase in the coming years. The documentation and related coverage criteria go hand in hand, and their importance cannot be overstated. Effective documentation assists in meeting patients' needs and may assist in safe-guarding team members from Medicare fraud or abuse claims. Quality documentation also assists in reimbursement for appropriate, medically necessary, covered hospice services. Clinical documentation continues to be an important indicator of the quality of care provided in hospice care. Documentation helps ensure that patients and families are receiving medically necessary, appropriate, and high-quality hospice care. With the move toward paying for quality care, hospice team members all have an important part to play in care and its documentation. By telling their patient's story through the hospice documentation, hospice nurses and other team members play a crucial role in the lives of patients and fami-lies and communities every day.

## References

Buerhaus, P. I., Auerbach, D. I., & Staiger, D. O. (2009). The recent surge in nurse employment: Causes and implications. *HealthAffairs, 28*(4), w657–w668.

Centers for Medicare and Medicaid Services. (2008). Medicare and Medicaid programs: Hospice conditions of participation. Retrieved from https://www.gpo.gov/fdsys/pkg/FR-2008-06-05/pdf/08-1305.pdf

CGS. (2013, Oct 28a). Hospice documentation. Retrieved from https://www.cgsmedicare.com/hhh/education/materials/pdf/hospice_clinical_factors_recert_tool.pdf

CGS. (2013, Oct 28b). Suggestions for improved documentation to support Medicare hospice services. Retrieved from http://www.cgsmedicare.com/hhh/education/materials/pdf/hospice_documentation_tool.pdf

Grant, R. (2016, Feb 3). The U.S. is running out of nurses. Retrieved from https://www.theatlantic.com/health/archive/2016/02/nursing-shortage/459741/

The National Academies Press Open Book. (2011). The future of nursing: Leading change, advancing health. Retrieved from http://www.nap.edu/read/12956/chapter/1

National Hospice and Palliative Care Organization. (2010, Nov 2). Retrieved from https://www.nhpco.org/sites/default/files/public/regulatory/FacetoFace.pdf

# Planning, Managing, and Coordinating Care

Hospice care is individualized by the interdisciplinary group (IDG) for each patient and the patient's family. Needs are assessed through an initial and comprehensive assessment process, and the IDG develops a plan of care (POC) to meet those needs. The assessment and care planning processes are continuous and overlapping and depend on the IDG's planning and coordination of care skills. This part discusses the comprehensive assessment and the POC as it relates to planning, management, and coordination of care for the hospice patient and the family.

## THE HOSPICE INITIAL AND COMPREHENSIVE ASSESSMENT

The initial and comprehensive assessments are the drivers for all care and care planning. The following information will help to delineate the difference and the important data needed for these requirements.

### INITIAL ASSESSMENT

To deliver the right care to the patient and family, there must first be an assessment by the hospice IDG. An RN has 48 hours from the effective date of the hospice election to complete an initial assessment of the patient's needs. The regulatory requirements for the initial and comprehensive assessment are contained in the Medicare hospice Conditions of Participation (CoPs) at §418.54 Condition of Participation: Initial and Comprehensive Assessment of the Patient. The purpose of this initial assessment is to collect the information necessary to treat the patient's/family's immediate care needs in the location where the patient will receive hospice care. The regulations specify that the RN must be the first to begin the assessment process for the IDG (Centers for Medicare and Medicaid Services [CMS], 2008).

An initial RN assessment works well when there is a short window of time to determine the pressing needs of the patient. Generally, an initial assessment takes place in a shorter time than a comprehensive assessment, and the RN communicates and coordinates with the patient's attending physician and hospice physician about the patient's priority needs and interventions for symptom management (CMS, 2008). Examples of this situation could be when a patient is discharged from the hospice late in the day and is too tired for a long admission visit. The RN would assess and meet the patient's immediate needs and plan to return the next day to complete a more in-depth nursing assessment of the patient's/family's needs and to begin developing the POC. Another example of the initial assessment being appropriate is a patient who is referred to hospice care when he or she is imminently dying. In this situation, the RN is assessing the patient's urgent needs to provide care that enhances comfort and maintains dignity. Depending on the patient's status, the rest of the IDG may not be able to complete a comprehensive assessment before the patient dies. If that happens, the IDG members who were not able to complete their assessment would document in the clinical record that they could not complete it because of the patient's imminent death.

## COMPREHENSIVE ASSESSMENT

An RN is required to visit the patient before other members of the IDG to begin the comprehensive assessment of the patient's/family's needs. The IDG has 5 calendar days from the effective date of the hospice election to complete an assessment of the patient's/family's physical, emotional, psychosocial, and spiritual needs. The patient and family have the right to refuse specific services, such as spiritual services, but the refusal of a service does not preclude the IDG from assessing the patient's/family's needs in that area (CMS, 2008). For example, the patient and family may prefer to interact with the spiritual counselor from their church instead of the hospice spiritual professional. That is fine, but assessment of spiritual needs must still be documented in the clinical record as well as the plan for meeting those needs in the patient's POC. The hospice spiritual professional would remain involved as part of the IDG team to lend expertise and guidance to the team as necessary. The comprehensive assessment screens physical problems, mental status, emotional distress, spiritual needs, support systems, and family needs for counseling and education. The specific content includes the requirement to document the patient status related to the following:

- Pain and severity of symptoms
- Nature and condition causing admission (terminality)
- Complications and risk factors that affect care planning
- Functional status, including the patient's ability to understand and participate in his or her own care
- Imminence of death
- Drug profile
- Initial bereavement status and needs
- Need for referrals and further evaluation by applicable health professionals (CMS, 2008)

A hospice may choose its own assessment form or tool, but the components and content of the assessment must include those specified in §418.54 Condition of Participation: Initial and Comprehensive Assessment of the Patient. (See components of the Hospice CoPs in Appendix A and B.) The comprehensive assessment may involve several forms, which is acceptable. A hospice organization should document the names of the forms that comprise the comprehensive assessment in its comprehensive assessment policy. The hospice IDG is also required to document an update of the comprehensive assessment in the clinical record no less frequently than every 15 days or as frequently as the patient status requires an update. The updates to the comprehensive assessment can be in any format the hospice chooses, but they must be clearly labeled as the update to the comprehensive assessment in the clinical record (CMS, 2008).

The comprehensive assessment is the vehicle for the collection of clinical information the hospice physician uses to determine the terminal diagnosis and diagnoses that contribute to the terminal prognosis. *When the patient was referred and admitted to hospice (meaning where in the disease trajectory continuum) influences relatedness of a diagnosis to the terminal prognosis.* For example, Mr. Jones has a terminal diagnosis of prostate cancer, but he also has a history of diabetes. At the time of his admission, 3 months before his death, the hospice physician determined that the diabetes did not contribute to the terminal prognosis. But because Mr. Jones's cancer advanced and his physical status declined, the hospice physician determined that diabetes was now related; therefore, hospice managed the diagnosis and covered its associated cost.

The comprehensive assessment provides the content for the patient's POC, which is the roadmap for the IDG to provide hospice care. The link between these two tools is direct and critical as one feeds the other. Since the introduction of the initial and comprehensive assessment CoP in the 2008 Medicare CoPs, different standards under this CoP have consistently been included in the Centers for Medicare and Medicaid Services' (CMS) top 10 survey deficiencies, which are updated annually. Compliance with the time frame of the comprehensive assessment has been the most cited by CMS since 2008. The regulation states that the comprehensive assessment should be completed no later than 5 calendar days after the effective date of hospice election (CMS, 2008). For example, if the patient's election for hospice is effective on Monday, then the hospice has until the following Saturday (which is 5 calendar days after Monday) to complete the comprehensive assessment.

# THE HOSPICE PLAN OF CARE AND COORDINATION OF CARE

CMS considers the plan of care (POC) to be the most important document in hospice care, and its requirements are outlined in the Medicare CoPs at §418.56 Condition of Participation: Interdisciplinary Group, Care Planning, and Coordination of Services. The POC is the roadmap for the IDG to provide interventions that address the physical, emotional, psychosocial, and spiritual problems of the patient and family. The hospice team is interdisciplinary, meaning that all the team members are working toward the same goals. The required, or "core," interdisciplinary group members include:

- A hospice physician
- A registered nurse
- A social worker
- A spiritual counselor
- A dietary counselor (as needed)

The development of the POC is not accomplished in an IDG vacuum; rather, it includes the input of both the patient and the family as well the patient's attending physician. Documentation by the IDG in the clinical record should reflect the patient's/family's level of understanding, involvement, and agreement with the POC, in accordance with the hospice's policies and the requirements in the Medicare CoPs. The IDG should also be developing a patient's POC proactively by anticipating patient changes and needs. For example, ordering an opioid for pain will most likely cause constipation, so a laxative is proactively ordered simultaneously with the opioid to avoid this outcome. IDG care planning incorporates decisions to avoid crises and reflects the patient/family preferences (CMS, 2008).

The POC is always changing and should not be viewed as a static process that is only addressed at designated regulatory time points. The POC identifies the hospice care and services necessary to meet the patient- and family-specific needs that are identified in the comprehensive assessment as it relates to the terminal illness and related conditions. There is a link between the assessed patient and family needs in the comprehensive assessment and the POC that the hospice IDG develops. The IDG is responsible for including services and treatments in the POC that are related to the terminal illness and related conditions, even if the hospice identified other needs in the patient assessment that are not related to the terminal prognosis. The IDG should use the POC as a tool to ensure that all team members are coordinated in relation to the care interventions for the patient and family (CMS, 2008).

Medicare regulations require the hospice to develop a process of communication, coordination, supervision, and integration related to the patient's POC. The process should be outlined in a hospice policy/procedure, and practice should follow the policy. Although the regulations do not specify the manner in which the IDG coordinates and updates the patient's POC, hospice industry best practice is to facilitate a weekly IDG meeting to discuss updates to the patient's comprehensive assessment and POC. This is the time when all team members share pertinent information about the patient's/family's status, progress toward current goals, and development of new goals as necessary. Coordination ensures that the IDG provides care and services in accordance with the POC and based on the patient's/family's assessed needs at any given time. In addition to coordinating care within the IDG for all diagnoses that contribute to the terminal prognosis, the hospice must share information with other nonhospice healthcare providers who are furnishing services unrelated to the terminal prognosis. This coordination of care must be documented clearly in the clinical record (CMS, 2008).

The RN is designated as the manager of the POC per the CoPs. The RN is a member of the IDG and provides POC coordination to ensure continuous assessment of the patient's and family's needs and implementation of the interdisciplinary POC, which includes collaboration with the patient's attending physician, the patient or representative, and family (CMS, 2008). The content of a patient's hospice POC is individualized but must include the following content:

- **Interventions to manage pain and symptoms**—There should be evidence in the clinical record that the IDG addresses the patient's symptoms, such as pain, nausea, vomiting, dehydration, constipation, dyspnea, emotional distress, and spiritual needs, using accepted professional standards of practice.

- **The scope and frequency of services necessary to meet the individualized patient and family needs**—There is no rubric or guide for hospice visits; the number of visits for any member of the IDG is determined based on the patient's/family's assessed needs. The Medicare CoPs allow individual visit ranges as long as they are small (one to two visits/week). The number of visits in the range may be exceeded by the IDG to address patient's/family's needs. In that instance, there should be documentation in the clinical record to explain the need for the extra visit(s).

  - **Physician orders for visits**—These should be obtained for nurses and social workers; the IDG supervises and approves visit frequency for spiritual counselors and volunteers.

  - **Missed visits**—No physician order should be required for a missed visit, but if the visit frequency must be changed, a physician order is recommended for nurses and social workers; the IDG supervises and approves visit frequency for spiritual counselors and volunteers.

  - **PRN ("as needed") visits**—PRN visits are visits that are provided as the patient's status requires and are viewed as "extra" visits to an established visit frequency. PRN visits may be included as an addition to an established visit frequency to ensure the most appropriate level of service is provided to the patient. However, if the patient requires frequent use of PRN visits, the POC visit frequency should be increased to include the need for additional visits. Although the Medicare regulations do not specify that the PRN visit number and reason be documented in the POC, including this detail truly individualizes the patient's POC. PRN should never be used as a stand-alone visit frequency for any discipline.

- **Standing orders**—Standing orders or routine orders are allowable, but they must be individualized to address the specific patient's needs and be signed by the patient's attending physician (CMS, 2008).

> **NOTE** Hospice organizations should check their state hospice licensure regulations and accreditation standards (as applicable) to assess whether stricter guidance is in place related to the scope and frequency of services. Should there be a question related to your state hospice licensure or other regulations, see Appendix C for your state hospice association.

- **Measurable outcomes**—A patient's POC must have outcomes for the patient and family that are measurable as a result of the implementation of the POC. The IDG should also be using data elements in the POC as a benchmark to determine whether they are meeting the goals of care (CMS, 2008). For example, a patient with pain describes the intensity of the pain as 7 out of 10 on a pain measurement scale of 0–10. An opioid is prescribed by the physician to control the pain, and the patient states that he would like to achieve a pain score of 4 out of 10 within 7 days of beginning opioid therapy. This is a clear and measurable goal. Documentation in the clinical record should indicate the patient's/family's participation in goal formation, IDG interventions for goal attainment, and the patient's/family's progress toward goal achievement.

- **Drugs and treatment**—Every patient has a right to receive effective pain management and symptom control from the hospice IDG related to all diagnoses that contribute to the terminal prognosis. All drugs and treatments for pain and symptom control must be included on the patient's POC (CMS, 2008).

- **Medical supplies and equipment necessary to meet the needs of the patient**—The hospice must provide all supplies and durable medical equipment related to all diagnoses that contribute to the terminal prognosis that are necessary and reasonable to meet the needs of the patient (CMS, 2008).

## REVIEW OF THE PLAN OF CARE

The Medicare hospice regulations require the hospice IDG, in collaboration with the patient's attending physician (if any), to review and revise a patient's individualized POC as frequently as the patient's condition requires, but no less frequently than every 15 calendar days. Communication with the attending physician may be accomplished via phone calls, electronic methods, or other means according to hospice policy and per patient needs. All members of the hospice team should be able to describe the care plan review process and how collaboration occurs among the IDG and the patient's attending physician. The revised POC must include updated information from the updated comprehensive assessment and indicate the patient's progress toward the specified goals of care. Any update to the patient's POC should be shared with all IDG members at the time of update. Documentation of communication with IDG members regarding updates to the patient's POC outside of an IDG meeting should be documented in the clinical record (CMS, 2008).

## MEDICATION MANAGEMENT

Managing the patient's medication is a care planning process that begins at the time of the comprehensive assessment and ends with the patient's death or discharge. It is critical for the RN to assess and reconcile all medications the patient is taking at the time of admission and on every visit thereafter. Some patients hold on to expired medication for years, so assessing and assisting the patient with disposal of expired medications is part of the medication management process. The RN is required to review all prescription and over-the-counter drugs, herbal remedies, and other alternative treatments that could affect drug therapy. The RN must identify:

- The effectiveness of drug therapy
- Drug side effects
- Actual or potential drug interactions
- Duplicate drug therapy
- Drug therapy currently associated with laboratory monitoring

In addition, the hospice should consider the use of pharmacological and nonpharmacological interventions to promote the patient's comfort level and sense of well-being based on the assessment of patient needs and desires (CMS, 2008).

Medication assessment and management also includes a review of medications that are no longer medically necessary for the patient at that point in the disease trajectory. The hospice physician reviews all medications for medical necessity and recommends the discontinuance of medications that are deemed no longer medically necessary. Decreasing medications can be beneficial to the patient because it can reduce daily pill burden and polypharmacy, which can promote comfort. The patient and family also need to receive an understandable explanation from the hospice physician or RN related to why the patient no longer needs a specific medication. If it is the patient's and family's desire for the patient to continue taking a medication that is not medically necessary for the palliation of the terminal illness, it is okay to do so, but neither hospice nor any other part of Medicare will pay for it.

Maintaining an accurate drug profile is a crucial part of the medication management process. Ensuring that all medications are on the profile and that the profile in the patient's home matches the profile in the clinical record is a continuous process for the RN. The RN should ask the patient and family the following questions on every nursing visit:

> "Was there a change to your medications since my last visit?"

> "Did you add or discontinue any medications since my last visit?"

The medication profile is the comprehensive overview to the patient's medication regimen. Accuracy is everything in this area of care.

 **NOTE** The Food and Drug Administration (FDA) regards oxygen to be a prescription drug, so it must have a physician order, and it must appear on the medication profile (FDA, 2016).

The hospice team should be alert to assess patient reaction to controlled medications because they can increase risk for falls. When a patient is prescribed a controlled medication for symptom control, the team should automatically include a fall assessment and fall precautions into the patient's plan of care.

## CONTROLLED DRUG MANAGEMENT AND DISPOSAL

Hospice team members should *not* carry medications on their person or in their vehicles. Several factors contribute to this, not the least of which is potential violations of federal or state dispensing laws, and potential diversion or allegations of diversion.

As of October 2014, a law from the Drug Enforcement Administration (DEA) prohibits hospice staff from actively wasting or destroying the patient's controlled drugs at the time of death. The DEA states that the drugs are the property of the patient and then become the property of the patient's family after death. Hospice staff may educate family members about safe drug disposal and assist them in disposing of the medications, but they may not actively do the disposing (Department of Justice, 2014). Hospice providers should follow state and federal laws for drug disposal for noncontrolled drugs.

Since the CMS update to the CoPs in 2008, the initial and comprehensive assessment and the POC have consistently appeared in the top 10 Medicare recertification survey deficiencies for hospice providers. Areas of recurrent citation include timing of the assessment completion and inadequate or missing assessment content. From a compliance perspective, deficiencies in the IDG's assessment process will result in survey deficiencies and could impact the outcomes of a reimbursement audit. From a quality of care perspective, deficiencies in the IDG's assessment process impact how patient's/family's needs are assessed and met, which affect overall patient and caregiver satisfaction. The "Patient-Related Considerations" sidebar outlines these patient/family needs.

## PATIENT-RELATED CONSIDERATIONS

The following is a list of the most common patient-related considerations a clinician evaluates when formulating plans and beginning care. This alphabetical list is not all-inclusive; other considerations may apply, such as the hospice patient caseload and availability of services or other resources. Many of these factors are interrelated.

Absence of caregiver
Activities of daily living (ADL) limitations
Adaptive or assistive devices
Behavioral or mental disorders
Belief systems
Caregiver support/willingness/ availability
Chemical or drug problems (for example, alcoholism)
Chronic illness(es)
Clinician assessment and reassessment findings
Clinician diagnoses
Cognitive function
Communication
Compliance/noncompliance
Coping skills
Culture
Directives
Disabilities
Discharge plan
Educational level/barriers
Emergency plan
Environment of care
Family
Fatigue
Functional limitations

Goals/expected outcomes
Health literacy (patient/family)
History
Home medical equipment (in place and needs)
Independence
Instrumental activities of daily living (IADLs)
Knowledge of emergency procedures
Language barriers
Learning needs
Loss of significant other
Medications (number, type, interactions)
Mobility
Mood (for example, grief, depression, loneliness)
Motivation
Nutritional status
Orthotic needs
Pain
Parenting
Pathology
Physical assessment findings
Polypharmacy
Potential for further complications

| | |
|---|---|
| Prognosis | Self-care status |
| Psychopathology | Skin integrity |
| Psychosocial needs | Social factors |
| Reason for hospice referral | Social supports |
| Reason for prior hospitalizations | Socioeconomic condition |
| | Spiritual comfort/needs |
| Rehabilitative needs | Stability |
| Resources (for example, financial, human) | Support system |
| | Swallowing |
| Rights | Symptom management |
| Risk factors | Values |
| Safety | Voice |

# PATIENT DEATH

The patient's POC is individualized to provide interventions for comfort and quality of life with the goal of a peaceful death. The RN visits the patient and family at the time of death for the purposes of:

- Pronouncing death (nurses should check their state regulations for death pronouncement guidance)
- Contacting the hospice physician for a certification of death
- Comforting family members
- Providing education and assistance with drug disposal
- Contacting the funeral home for body pickup

A social worker or spiritual care counselor may be needed or requested on death visits depending on the family's needs and wishes. The hospice team should be aware of and honor any death rituals or ceremonies the family wants to commence at the time of the patient's death.

# CARE PLANNING AND IDG CULTURAL COMPETENCY

The end-of-life process is a momentous experience for a patient and family, and it can be challenging for the IDG to individualize care related to the cultural and religious beliefs of today's diverse population. A hospice team member's challenges can be further influenced by the amount of training and experience in cultural diversity and his or her comfort level in discussing the topic.

Cultural competency can be characterized as continual active engagement through the process of cultural awareness, cultural knowledge, cultural skills, cultural collaboration, and cultural encounters. Cultural awareness and competency of the IDG ensures the provision of individualized hospice care within the cultural context of the patient (Coolen, 2012).

The IDG must have sufficient knowledge, understanding, and recognition of the specific influences that culture has on a patient's and family's behavior, attitudes, preferences, and decisions related to end-of-life care. One cannot make assumptions about a patient's/family's beliefs; it is important to determine through assessment and conversation what their beliefs are and how they will affect the POC. Cultural and religious beliefs could affect symptom management, communication, and the disposition of the patient's body at the time of death. Assessment of cultural and religious beliefs should be part of the comprehensive assessment for the IDG and guide the collaborative care planning process between the IDG, the patient, and the family (Coolen, 2012).

# CASE STUDY: ELIGIBILITY AND THE PLAN OF CARE

Mr. Walsh is a 72-year old male who has the diagnosis of congestive heart failure, coronary artery disease, and ischemic cardiomyopathy. He is cared for at home by his wife, who is 70 years old and in fairly good health. Mr. Walsh had five hospitalizations for symptom exacerbations in the past year, which has caused loss of independence in activities of daily living, episodes of syncope, decreased appetite and ambulation, increased shortness of breath, and generalized weakness and debilitation. He has gained 15–20 pounds in the past 2 months, which has limited his activity to going from the bed to the chair or the commode chair. Mr. Walsh is prescribed 2 liters of oxygen. He has shortness of breath, intermittent chest pain (5 out of 10 on a 0–10 pain measurement scale) upon moderate exertion that is relieved with rest and nitroglycerin, 2+ pitting edema in bilateral lower extremities, a cardiac ejection fraction score of 35%, and a Palliative Performance Scale (PPS) score of 30. Mr. Walsh is not medically eligible for any aggressive treatments or surgery, and his physician has been managing his symptoms through drug therapy.

Mrs. Walsh has taken excellent care of her husband, but they both believe they need additional help because Mr. Walsh's condition is deteriorating. Both Mr. and Mrs. Walsh want to keep him at home, comfortable, with the best quality of life possible, and to avoid further hospitalizations in the future. They are people of faith and receive support from their local church in the form of parish visitors, visits from their minister, and occasional potluck deliveries. Mr. Walsh appears downhearted and withdrawn and has verbalized his fear about dying and leaving his wife alone.

1. Is Mr. Walsh eligible for hospice care? Why?

   Although the hospice physician makes the determination of eligibility, Mr. Walsh has been referred at the right time in his disease trajectory for hospice evaluation. His frequent hospitalizations in the past year, his weight gain, and his PPS score of 30 indicate the progression of his disease and his decline and appropriateness for a hospice evaluation.

2. The hospice physician determined that Mr. Walsh is eligible for hospice services. The hospice interdisciplinary hospice team completed a comprehensive assessment, and Mr. Walsh's POC was developed. What considerations does the team need to address in the POC?

The following issues should be addressed in Mr. Walsh's initial POC and in updates to his POC as long as they remain problems:

- Pain management
- Other symptom management (SOB, syncope, edema, weakness, weight gain)
- Functionality (ability to perform ADLs, ambulation)
- Safety (Mr. Walsh is a fall risk related to his syncope, weakness, SOB, edema, and pain medication)

3. What do you identify as the main goals in Mr. Walsh's POC?

The following would be important to address in the goals of care for Mr. Walsh. Goals should be measureable:

- Management of the disease process in the patient's location of choice, his home.
- Medication management. (The hospice physician recommends that Mr. Walsh discontinue taking his statin drugs because they are no longer medically necessary at this stage of his disease.)
- Pain management. (The goal should be developed based on what Mr. Walsh wants his pain level to be.)
- Shortness of breath management. (The goal should be developed based on what Mr. Walsh wants his comfort level to be.)
- Measures for reduction of syncope and edema.
- Fall safety measures and education for the patient and family.
- Social work intervention for counseling related to Mr. Walsh's emotional state and planning for post death.
- Spiritual care coordination with Mr. Walsh's minister directed toward life closure and support for the patient and family.

# CASE STUDY: FREQUENCY AND INTENSITY OF SERVICES

The following is an example of a patient and patient problem seen in hospice. This is *just* an example for discussion and review purposes. The hospice nurse's professional judgment, recognized standards of care, and information gathered from all aspects of the assessment process are the basis for identifying patient and family services, visit frequency, and service duration needs. All hospice documentation must clearly show the disease progression of the terminally ill patient.

The patient is a 47-year-old woman with cancer of the liver who is admitted for hospice care. The hospice clinical specialist, who admits the patient and family to the program, explains the hospice philosophy and proposes a care regimen based on the needs identified. Healthcare, home health aide care, and other components of the hospice team are explained, and care is scheduled to begin. The frequency issue is sometimes more complex in patients with clearly shortened life spans.

The answers to the following questions may help the hospice nurse determine the frequency and the intensity of hospice services. Determinations must be based on the patient's and family's unique findings, situation, and supports. Generally, hospice patients may have more intensive needs toward the end of care than at the beginning. This situation is the opposite of the typical home health case scenario, in which the patient is working toward independence and the team pulls back toward discharge. Keep in mind, however, that some patients are admitted to hospice appropriately for intensive services at the onset for hospice's specialty skills of support and pain and symptom management.

1. Why were the patient and family referred to hospice? Can hospice meet their unique needs?

2. What information has the doctor, patient, or others provided that supports the contention that the patient has a limited life expectancy?

3. What symptoms or clinical information supports the need for hospice?

4. What is the patient's current activity level, how has it changed, and how rapidly has it changed?

5. If this is a new diagnosis, what services are identified during the assessment, and how do these services support fulfillment of the patient and family needs?

6. If the patient has Alzheimer's disease, cardiac or lung disease, or another illness that may have long-term or chronic disease implications, what occurrences or symptoms lead the physician and clinicians to believe that the patient is dying?

7. Are symptoms or side effects from therapy emerging in the history and physical assessment?

8. What are the expectations related to hospice care and support, and how can they best be met?

9. What are the special skills and services that hospice will bring to this patient and family?

10. What are the patient and family expressing/identifying as their needs?

## SUMMARY

Through the process of comprehensive assessment, the IDG is able to determine the patient's and family's needs and build an individualized POC. The patient and family are the unit of care in hospice, and their wishes for a meaningful and comfortable end-of-life experience are achieved through the care planning process that involves the patient, the family, and the IDG. Significant components of the patient's POC are medication management and developing interventions that are culturally respectful and effective. The hospice journey begins with an assessment of the patient/family needs by the IDG and ends with the IDG at the family's side to help them cope with their loved one's death and assist them with the logistical issues associated with patient death.

# References

Centers for Medicare and Medicaid Services. (2008). Medicare and Medicaid programs: Hospice conditions of participation. Retrieved from https://www.gpo.gov/fdsys/pkg/FR-2008-06-05/pdf/08-1305.pdf

Coolen, P. R. (2012, May 1). Cultural relevance in end-of-life care. Retrieved from https://ethnomed.org/clinical/end-of-life/cultural-relevance-in-end-of-life-care

Department of Justice. (2014). Disposal of controlled substances: Final rule. Retrieved from https://www.deadiversion.usdoj.gov/fed_regs/rules/2014/2014-20926.pdf

Food and Drug Administration. (2016, Apr 13). Important Alert 66-37. Retrieved from https://www.accessdata.fda.gov/cms_ia/importalert_187.html

# Hospice Diagnoses and Guidelines for Care

Prior parts of this book addressed that the Medicare Hospice Benefit is prognosis-based, which means that the patient must have a limited life expectancy, and the hospice is responsible for caring for and covering all cost for the terminal or primary diagnosis and all diagnoses that contribute to the terminal prognosis. The benefit covers services, drugs, supplies, and medical equipment related to the terminal diagnosis and diagnoses that contribute to the terminal prognosis. The hospice physician determines which diagnosis is the primary one and which comorbidities contribute to the terminal prognosis by reviewing all available clinical information from the referral source and outcomes from the interdisciplinary comprehensive assessment. Determining relatedness of diseases to the terminal diagnosis is a complex process, so it is extremely important for the hospice physician to have as much information about the patient as possible. Determining relatedness is not a one-time event; it is a continuous process that begins at admission and continues throughout the hospice service period. A patient may have a disease process at the time of admission that does not contribute to the terminal prognosis, but as the disease progresses and the patient's status declines over time, that same disease process may contribute to the terminal prognosis and become the responsibility of the hospice interdisciplinary group (IDG) to manage.

The hospice IDG works together toward common goals determined by the patient, family, and IDG collaboratively. This means individualizing the care to manage the terminal diagnosis and diagnoses that contribute to the terminal prognosis. However, there are common symptoms at the end of life that a patient may experience no matter the specific diagnosis(es)—Table 4.1 outlines these common symptoms. A common goal is the preservation of quality of life and dignity for the patient. Adequately managing common symptoms at the end of life contributes to maintaining the quality of life the patient and family desires (National Cancer Institute, 2016).

**TABLE 4.1** Common Symptoms at the End of Life

| Symptom | Cause | Intervention |
|---|---|---|
| Fatigue | Progress of disease | Balance rest and activity for energy conservation |
| | Pain medication side effects | Medications that increase brain activity, alertness, and energy |
| | Coughing | |
| | Decreased food and fluid intake | |
| Anxiety | Pain | Medication to relieve anxiety |
| | Shortness of breath | Counseling to relieve psychosocial, emotional, or spiritual turmoil |
| | Psychosocial, emotional, or spiritual turmoil | Relaxation, breathing, and guided imagery exercises |
| Shortness of breath | Disease progression | Opioids to relieve shortness of breath in patients |
| | Excess fluid in the abdomen | Bronchodilators to relieve swelling and inflammation, which may relieve these spasms |
| | Loss of muscle strength | Increase in oxygen if shortness of breath is caused by hypoxemia |
| | | Cool fan placed toward the patient's face |

| Symptom | Cause | Intervention |
|---------|-------|--------------|
| Shortness of breath *(continued)* | Hypoxia/hypoxemia<br>Pneumonia<br>Infection | Having the patient sit up or prop to a 45-degree angle in bed<br>Teaching a patient to do breathing and relaxation exercises, if able<br>Consideration of antibiotics if shortness of breath is caused by an infection |
| Pain | Disease progression<br>Excess fluid in the abdomen<br>Shortness of breath<br>Coughing | Opioids to control pain at the end of life |
| Coughing | Excess fluid in the abdomen<br>Shortness of breath<br>Increased mucus<br>Difficulty in swallowing | Over-the-counter cough medications with expectorants to increase bronchial fluids and loosen mucus<br>Medications to decrease mucus<br>Opioids to stop the coughing |
| Constipation | Pain medication<br>Decreased food and fluid intake<br>Decreased activity | Laxative medication<br>Increased fluid intake<br>A laxative prescribed with opioid medication |
| Difficulty swallowing | Disease progression<br>Fatigue<br>Shortness of breath | Offering small amounts of food that the patient enjoys<br>Modifying food textures as needed (pureed, chopped, thickened)<br>Altering administration of medications from oral to other routes |
| Nausea and vomiting | Disease process<br>Medications<br>Pain<br>Sensitivity to smells, tastes, or sight of food | Medication to relieve nausea and pain<br>Management of patient environment to exclude triggers of nausea |

*(continues)*

**TABLE 4.1** Common Symptoms at the End of Life *(continued)*

| Symptom | Cause | Intervention |
|---|---|---|
| Decreased appetite | Nausea and vomiting | Changing or adjusting medication for symptom control |
| | Fatigue | |
| | Pain (physical, emotional, spiritual) | Adding nutritional supplements to diet |
| | A change in taste | Medication to stimulate appetite |
| | Loss of taste | |
| | Sensitivity to smells | |
| | Difficulty swallowing | |
| | Shortness of breath | |
| | Constipation or diarrhea | |
| | Medication for symptom control | |

(National Cancer Institute, 2016)

# COMMON SYMPTOMS IN THE LAST DAYS OF LIFE (ACTIVE DYING)

Active dying is the process by which the patient's body shuts down and death is expected to occur within days. (The days can vary with each patient.) Patients often experience a gradual decline in neurological, cognitive, cardiovascular, respiratory, gastrointestinal, genitourinary, and muscular function, which is typical of the dying process (National Cancer Institute, 2016). Table 4.2 outlines the common symptoms most patients experience during the last days of life.

**TABLE 4.2** Common Symptoms During Last Days of Life

| Symptom | Cause | Intervention |
|---|---|---|
| Changes in level of consciousness—increased sleep | Disease process | Patient rest |
| | Fatigue | Family support |
| | Medications | Meaningful activity and communication during wakeful periods |

| Symptom | Cause | Intervention |
| --- | --- | --- |
| Delirium and terminal restlessness | Direct effects of cancer or other causes such as these:<br><br>Disease process<br><br>Side effects of drugs or drug interactions<br><br>Metabolic imbalance<br><br>Dehydration<br><br>Untreated pain<br><br>Constipation<br><br>Fear, anxiety, or emotional turmoil | Evaluation and change (as needed) of pain and other symptom control medications<br><br>Treating dehydration through fluid administration<br><br>Treating constipation (laxatives or other interventions as appropriate)<br><br>Antianxiety medications<br><br>Palliative sedation related to the intensity of delirium and terminal restlessness |
| Pulselessness on the radial artery | Decreased circulation<br><br>Decreased intensity of blood circulation | Comfort measures such as adjusting patient position in bed |
| Decreased urine output | Decreased fluid intake<br><br>Decreased kidney function | Comfort measures such as offering sips of water (as able) and caring for the mouth to keep mucous membranes moist |
| Cheyne-Stokes breathing<br><br>Apnea periods | Decreased cardiopulmonary function | Comfort measures such as aiming a cool fan toward the patient's face or raising the patient's head position in bed |
| Rattling sound with breathing | Saliva or other fluids building up in the throat and airways in a patient who is too weak to cough | Medications to decrease the amount of saliva in the mouth or to dry the upper airway<br><br>Raising the head of the bed or propping the patient with pillows<br><br>Turning the patient to either side<br><br>Gentle suctioning (per the patient's tolerance) |

*continues*

**TABLE 4.2** Common Symptoms at End of Life *(continued)*

| Symptom | Cause | Intervention |
|---|---|---|
| Mottled skin, cold extremities | Decreased cardiopulmonary function | Comfort measures such as placing a heavier blanket on the patient or gently rubbing the patient's extremities |
| Changes in expression and special requests | Approaching death | Listening to and acknowledging patient's communication<br><br>Attempting to fulfill special requests |

(National Cancer Institute, 2016)

# STAGING SCALES

Various scales assess patient function, but the two scales that are used most commonly by hospice and palliative care professionals are the Palliative Performance Scale (PPS) and the Karnofsky Performance Scale (KPS).

- The Palliative Performance Scale (PPS) is a tool used by hospice and palliative care professionals to measure progressive patient decline. The scale has five functional dimensions:

  1. Ambulation

  2. Activity level and evidence of disease

  3. Self-care

  4. Oral intake

  5. Level of consciousness

  The tool has 11 defined levels of PPS, from 0% to 100% in 10% increments. Every decrease in 10% marks a fairly significant decrease in physical function. Determining a patient's PPS score serves as a way for the IDG to determine patient function status. It is important that clinicians be trained to administer the scale and the scale instructions are followed to ensure accurate assessment (Anderson, Downing, Hill, Casorso, & Lerch, 1995).

- The Karnofsy Performance Scale (KPS) is a tool that measures the ability of a patient to perform activities of daily living (ADLs) and can also be used for prognostic purposes. The KPS scores range from 0 to 10, and the higher the score, the better a patient can carry out daily activities (Schag, Heinrich, & Ganz, 1984).

# GUIDELINES FOR HOSPICE CARE

The next section outlines common hospice diagnoses by system and provides care guidance for each core team member of the hospice IDG. Some members of the hospice team are designated as noncore, or their intervention occurs after the patient's death. Their care guidance is outlined in the following sections.

## VOLUNTEER(S)

- Support, friendship, companionship, and presence
- Errands and transportation
- Other services, based on interdisciplinary group recommendations and patient/caregiver needs

## DIETITIAN/NUTRITIONAL COUNSELING

- Assessment of patient with cachexia and nausea
- Assessment and recommendations for swallowing difficulties
- Teaching and support of family members and caregivers
- Support and care with food and nourishment as desired by patient
- Assessment of family's view of benefits/burdens of tube feeding to prolong life

## OCCUPATIONAL THERAPIST

- Evaluation of activities of daily living (ADLs) and functional mobility
- Assess need for adaptive equipment and assistive devices

- Safety assessment of patient's environment and ADLs
- Assessment for energy conservation training

## PHYSICAL THERAPY

- Evaluation
- Safety assessment of patient's environment
- Instructing and supervising caregivers and volunteers on home exercise program/range of motion (ROM) and safe transfers

## BEREAVEMENT COUNSELOR

- Assessment of the needs of the bereaved family and friends
- Support and intervention, based on assessment and ongoing findings
- Presence and counseling
- Supportive visits and follow-up, other interventions (for example, mailings, calls)
- Services related to bereavement work and support

## COMPLEMENTARY THERAPIES

- Assessment plan to engage patient and support comfort, quality, enjoyment, and dignity
- Therapeutic touch therapy as requested by patient and family (for example, massage, reiki)
- Music therapy intervention based on assessment to decrease pain and other symptom perception
- Emotional support and expression
- Improved comfort and relaxation
- Maintenance of patient's comfort, physical, psychosocial, emotional, and spiritual health
- Pet therapy (including patient's pet, if available) and therapeutic intervention

# ALZHEIMER'S DISEASE AND OTHER DEMENTIAS CARE

## 1. GENERAL CONSIDERATIONS

As the baby boomer population ages and increasing numbers of elderly patients are cared for by their families or other caregivers in the home, the presence of Alzheimer's disease, organic brain syndrome, and other problems characterized by confusion continues to rise. The skills of the hospice team are important to ensuring the care and safety of these patients and their families. Patients with Alzheimer's disease and other dementias may be appropriate candidates for hospice care in their final stages. Compassion and care are then directed toward comfort and support of the patient and family or caregivers.

## 2. ELIGIBILITY CONSIDERATIONS

Patient eligibility for hospice is determined by the hospice physician in consultation with the referring and/or patient's attending physician. The Medicare Administrative Contractor (MAC) hospice local coverage determinations (LCDs) for Alzheimer's disease should be used by the physician and hospice team when making the eligibility determination. The LCDs state the following related to hospice eligibility for Alzheimer's disease:

> "The identification of specific structural/functional impairments, together with any relevant activity limitations, should serve as the basis for palliative interventions and care planning. The structural and functional impairments associated with a primary diagnosis of Alzheimer's disease are often complicated by comorbid and/or secondary conditions. Comorbid conditions affecting beneficiaries with Alzheimer's disease are by definition, distinct from the Alzheimer's disease itself; examples include coronary heart disease (CHD) and chronic obstructive pulmonary disease (COPD). Secondary conditions

on the other hand are directly related to a primary condition—in the case of Alzheimer's disease examples include delirium and pressure ulcers" (Palmetto GBA, 2017).

When addressing Alzheimer's disease and other dementias, refer to your MAC or other regulatory bodies for up-to-date and specific guidance.

## 3. POTENTIAL DIAGNOSES ICD-10-CM DIAGNOSTIC CODING

The *International Statistical Classification of Diseases and Related Health Problems* 10th Revision (ICD-10-CM) is a coding of diseases and signs, symptoms, abnormal findings, complaints, social circumstances, and external causes of injury or diseases, as classified by the WHO. There are specific coding rules and conventions in the official coding manual that must be followed, and these rules may not be included in online websites or EMR software. Consult with a credentialed coder for any questions related to accurate coding.

Dementia codes are listed in Chapter V: "Mental and Behavioral Disorders" and Chapter IV: "Diseases of the Nervous System" in the ICD-10-CM.

F01.50–F01.51 Vascular dementia

F03.90–F03.91 Unspecified dementia

F05 Delirium due to known physical condition

F06.0–F06.34, F06.8 Other mental disorders due to known physical condition

F07.0–F07.9 Personality/behavior disorders due to known physical condition

F09 Unspecified mental disorder

G30.0 Alzheimer's disease (use additional code to identify delirium if applicable with early onset)

G30.1 Alzheimer's disease with late onset

G31.83 Dementia with Lewy bodies, with Parkinsonism (F05), or dementia with behavioral disturbance (F02.81), or without behavioral disturbance (F02.80)

Z91.83 Use an additional code to identify wandering if applicable (see Chapter XXI)

The Centers for Medicare and Medicaid Services (CMS) issued Change Request 8877 on August 22, 2014, which listed multiple dementia diagnosis codes that cannot be used as the principal diagnosis according to ICD-10-CM Coding Guidelines. If any of the listed diagnoses are reported as a principal diagnosis, the hospice claim will be returned to the provider for a more definitive hospice diagnosis based on ICD-10-CM Coding Guidelines (CMS, 2014).

## 4. SAFETY CONSIDERATIONS

- Infection control and prevention/standard precautions
- Supervised medication administration
- Multiple medications safety (side effects, interactions, storage)
- Home medical equipment safety, including oxygen
- Nightlight
- Removal of scatter rugs
- Tub rail, grab bars for bathroom safety
- Supportive and nonskid shoes
- Smoking and oxygen safety
- Handrails on stairs
- Fall precautions
- Protective skin measures
- Stairway precautions
- Smoke detector and fire evacuation plan
- Assistance with ambulation
- Supervised care and medication regimen
- Others, based on the patient's unique condition and environment

## 5. SKILLS AND SERVICES IDENTIFIED

The Reisberg (1988) Functional Assessment Staging (FAST) Scale has been used for many years as a scale to assess patient function specific to Alzheimer's disease. The FAST Scale is a 16-item scale designed to parallel the progressive activity limitations associated with Alzheimer's disease. Stage 7 identifies the threshold of activity limitation that would support a 6-month prognosis in tandem with an assessment of comorbid conditions. The LCDs guide a clinician to look at the FAST score and the impact of comorbid and secondary conditions to assist in making a hospice eligibility determination.

It is important that clinicians be trained to administer the scale and that the scale instructions are followed to ensure an accurate assessment.

### Comorbid Conditions

The impact of comorbid conditions is best determined by defining the structural/functional impairments with any limitation in activity that is a result of, or related to, the comorbid condition.

Example: Alzheimer's disease and active CHD or COPD would have specific impairments of the cardiopulmonary system that may or may not respond to treatment. Clinicians would assess for dyspnea, orthopnea, wheezing, and chest pain. The impairments in cardiopulmonary function may be associated with activity limitations such as mobility and self-care. Ultimately, the combined effects of the Alzheimer's disease (FAST stage 7 and beyond) and any comorbid condition would most likely have a prognosis of 6 months or less (Palmetto GBA, 2017).

### Secondary Conditions

Alzheimer's disease may be complicated by secondary conditions. The occurrence of secondary conditions in patients with Alzheimer's disease is enabled by the presence of impairments in mental functioning and movement that can contribute to the increased incidence of secondary conditions such as delirium and pressure ulcers. The combined effects of the Alzheimer's disease (FAST stage 7 and beyond) and any secondary would most likely have a prognosis of 6 months or less (Palmetto GBA, 2017).

## Registered Nurse

### Comfort and Symptom Management

**Assess**

- Completing initial and comprehensive assessment of all systems of patient admitted to hospice for _____ (specify problem necessitating care)
- Assessing vital signs every visit
- Assessing patient, family, and caregiver wishes and expectations regarding care
- Assessing patient, family, and caregiver resources available for care
- Assessing pain and other symptoms, including site, duration, characteristics; evaluating the pain management's effectiveness; identifying need for change, addition, or other plan or dose adjustment

**Teach Patient and Family/Caregiver**

- Presenting of hospice philosophy and services
- Explaining patient rights and responsibilities
- Teaching physical care of patient
- Teaching about specific disease and management at end of life
- Teaching new pain and symptom control medication regimen
- Teaching symptom control and relief measures
- Teaching care of weak, terminally ill patient
- Instruction in pain control measures and medications
- Teaching about realistic expectations of disease process
- Teaching care of the dying and identifying signs/symptoms of impending death

**Provide Care/Case Management**

- Comprehensive care coordination with all members of the IDG and other healthcare providers
- Care plan oversight

- Skilled assessment and support of the patient, family, and caregiver's coping skills
- Medication management
- Home medical equipment as indicated
- Interventions of symptoms directed toward comfort and palliation
- Comfort measures of backrub and hand or other therapeutic massage
- Presence and support
- Volunteer support to patient and family per their request
- Other interventions, based on patient/family needs

### Safety and Mobility Considerations

- Providing caregiver with home safety information and instruction related to _____
- Teaching family regarding safety of patient in home
- Teaching family regarding energy conservation techniques
- Teaching safe oral intake (especially liquids)
- Monitoring for choking/aspiration if oral intake is possible
- Teaching caregiver safe and effective suctioning of patient secretions
- Teaching caregiver/family safety related to bed mobility and transfers
- Other interventions, based on patient/family needs

### Emotional/Spiritual Considerations

- Psychosocial assessment of patient and family regarding disease and prognosis (may be completed by the RN or the hospice social worker)
- Providing emotional support to patient and family with _____, and illness of a terminal nature
- Assessing mental status and sleep disturbance changes
- Assessing signs/symptoms of depression

- Spiritual counseling/support offered to patients and caregiver who verbalize emotional or spiritual pain and turmoil
- Providing support to patient and family/caregivers
- Other interventions, based on patient/family needs

### Skin Considerations

**Assess**

- Assessment and observation of skin integrity and patient's physical status
- Observation and assessment/evaluation of any wound and surrounding skin
- Evaluating patient's need for equipment/supplies to decrease pressure; alternating pressure mattress, gel foam seat cushion, and heel and elbow protectors
- Observing and applying skilled assessment of areas for possible breakdown, including bony prominences and other pressure-prone areas

**Teach Patient and Family/Caregiver**

- Skin care related to patient's needs, including the need for frequent position changes, appropriate pressure pads and mattresses, effective use of turn/pull sheet to avoid friction, skin tears and burns, and the prevention of breakdown
- Proper body alignment and positioning in bed to prevent skin tears from shearing skin

**Provide Care**

- Palliative wound care that focuses on relieving suffering and improving the patient's quality of life when the wound no longer responds to, or the patient can no longer tolerate, curative treatment; palliative wound care concentrates on symptom management, addressing the problems of infection, pain, wound odor, exudate, and decreased self-confidence in end-of-life care (Wound Source, 2017)

- Pressure ulcer care as indicated
  - Changing dressing at wound site using aseptic technique of _____ (define ordered care)
  - Culturing wound and urine and sending to lab (per physician order)
  - Consideration of RN enterostomal therapist to visit patient and evaluate wound for specific palliative care needs
- Other interventions, based on patient/family needs

**Elimination Considerations**

- Assessment of bowel regimen, and implementation of program as needed
- Monitoring bowel patterns, including frequency of bowel movements, and evaluation of bowel regimen (for example, stool softeners, laxatives, and dietary changes)
- Checking for and removing impaction per physician orders
- Teaching caregiver daily catheter care and equipment care and signs and symptoms that necessitate calling the hospice
- Changing catheter (specify type, size, and frequency) as indicated
- Assessing amount and frequency of urinary output
- Other interventions, based on patient/family needs

**Hydration/Nutrition**

- Assessment and monitoring of hydration/nutrition status
- Diet counseling for patient with cachexia
- Teaching family/caregivers proper care of the feeding tube
- Supporting nutrition/hydration by offering patient choice of favorite or desired foods or liquids
- Maintaining nutrition/hydration by offering patient high-protein diet and food of choice as tolerated
- Teaching patient and family to expect decreased nutritional and fluid intake as disease progresses

- Monitoring and recording weights as ordered
- Other interventions, based on patient/family needs

### Therapeutic/Medication Regimens

- Completion of an assessment and reconciliation of all patient pre-scriptions and over-the-counter drugs, herbal remedies, and other alternative treatments that could affect drug therapy, including, but not limited to, identification of the following:
  - Effectiveness of drug therapy
  - Drug side effects
  - Actual or potential drug interactions
  - Duplicate drug therapy
  - Drug therapy currently associated with laboratory monitoring
- Instruction on all medications including schedule, functions of specific drugs, and their side effects/interactions
- Monitoring and assessment of complications for new medication regimen
- Management of medications related to drug/drug, drug/food side effects
- Monitoring patient's response to medications for pain and symptom control
- Monitoring adherence to medication regimen
- Assessment of the patient's unique response to treatments or inter-ventions, and reporting changes or unfavorable responses or reac-tions to the physician
- Teaching new pain and symptom control medication regimen
- Teaching patient and family about new medications and side effects
- Obtaining venipuncture as ordered every _____ (order frequency)
- Teaching patient and caregiver use of patient-controlled analgesic (PCA) pump
- Assessment for electrolyte imbalance

- Nonpharmacological interventions such as progressive muscle relaxation, imagery, positive visualization, music, massage and touch, and humor therapy of patient's choice
- Other interventions, based on patient/family needs

### Other Considerations

- Assessment of disease progression
- Assistance to family in setting up patient-centered routine and stressing the importance of adhering to the routine once established
- Assessment of the patient's response to treatments and interventions and reporting to the physician any changes, unfavorable responses, or reactions
- Other interventions, based on patient/family needs

### Hospice Aide

- Effective and safe personal care
- Safe ADL assistance and support, ambulation, and transfers
- Observance of and reporting of any changes in patient condition
- Preparation or assistance with preparation of meals
- Homemaker services (as requested by family)
- Comfort care measures per patient needs and aide care plan
- Other duties as assigned and within the scope of practice

### Social Worker

- Completion of psychosocial assessment
- Support to patient and family/caregivers related to adjusting to the illness and its implications and the need for care
- Identification of optimal coping strategies
- Financial assessment and counseling regarding food acquisition and ability to prepare meals

- Interventions/support related to terminal illness and loss
- Emotional/spiritual support
- Facilitation of communication among patient, family, and hospice team
- Referrals/linkage to community services and resources as indicated
- Grief counseling and intervention/support related to illness/loss
- Identification of any illness-related psychiatric condition necessitating care
- Assistance with funeral and burial planning

## Volunteer(s)

- Support, friendship, companionship, and presence
- Comfort and dignity for patient and family
- Assistance with errands and transportation
- Other services based on interdisciplinary group recommendations and patient/caregiver needs

## Spiritual Counselor

- Spiritual assessment and care
- Counseling, interventions, and support related to life's meaning (consistent with patient's beliefs)
- Prayer with or for the patient's family using prayers familiar to patient's religious background (per their wishes)
- Support, listening, and presence
- Participation in sacred or spiritual rituals or practices
- Assistance with funeral planning
- Other supportive care, based on patient/family needs and belief systems

## 6. PATIENT, FAMILY, AND CAREGIVER EDUCATIONAL NEEDS

Educational needs are the care regimens that contribute to safe and effective care at home between the hospice team's visits. These include the following:

- The basic tenets of hospice and the availability of support 24 hours a day, 7 days a week
- Home safety assessment and counseling
- Safe and proper body mechanics to promote patient comfort and prevent caregiver safety problems
- Support groups available to the patient's family, such as caregiver support groups
- Skin care regimens
- Catheter and wound care programs
- Effective personal hygiene habits
- Home exercise program, including range of motion
- Safety measures in the home when the patient is immobilized
- Infection control and prevention
- Medication regimen and the medications' relationships to each other
- Importance of medical follow-up
- When to call the hospice
- Anticipated disease progression
- Other information based on the patient's/family's unique needs

## 7. TIPS FOR SUPPORTING QUALITY, SAFETY, AND ELIGIBILITY

- Know that the Medicare Hospice Benefit does not require that the patient be homebound or have identified skilled needs, but care must be medically necessary to qualify for Medicare reimbursement.

- Understand that, unless the patient has a hospice benefit, some insurers will not pay for a skilled nurse visit that is made at death if the patient is dead when the nurse arrives at the home.

- Should the patient's status deteriorate and increased personal care be needed, obtain a verbal order for the increased service, noting frequency and estimating the duration.

- Obtain a verbal order for all medication and skilled treatment changes (for example, antibiotic therapy), and document these in the clinical record.

- Document the symptoms and clinical assessment findings that support the terminal prognosis.

  - Patient changes, symptoms, and clinical information identified from visits and team meetings that support hospice care and limited life expectancy

    - Mentation, behavioral, and cognitive changes

    - Dysphagia, weight loss, dyspnea, infection, sepsis, and new or changed medications

    - Skin changes (for example, inflamed, painful, weeping skin site[s]) and reddened bony prominences

    - Dehydration

    - Patient change and decline

    - Pain, other symptoms not controlled

    - Status after acute episode of _____ (specify)

    - Positive urine, sputum culture; patient started

    - Febrile at _____, pulse change at _____, irregularly irregular

    - Medication adjustments

    - Nutrition, hydration, or elimination concerns (for example, decreased intake, fecal impaction)

    - Any variances to expected outcomes

- Inability to perform ADLs, personal care
- Frequent communication required with physician regarding _____ (specify)

- Clear support of the rationale that supports/explains the progression of the illness from the chronic to the terminal stages
- Coordination of services and consultations with other members of the IDG

- Document all IDG meetings and communications in the POC and in the progress notes of the clinical record.

- Document coordination of services or consultation providers, such as skilled nursing facility or nursing home staff, inpatient team members, and hired caregivers.

- Document what the patient looks like (frail, pale, poor intake, shortness of breath, inability to do ADLs, and so on).

- Ensure that all team members have provided input into the patient's POC and documented their interventions and goals.

- Remember that the clinical documentation is vital to measuring compliance for quality and reimbursement purposes. Care coordination, timely verbal and initial physician orders, and assessment and addressing of spiritual and psychosocial needs should be clearly documented in the patient's clinical record.

- Make sure the documentation supports that all hospice care is directed toward comfort and dignity while meeting patient/family needs.

- Ensure that all team members, including clinicians and social workers, assess, identify, and "hear" spiritual needs that the patient/family want to be addressed. These spiritual issues are important to the provision of quality hospice care and cannot be addressed effectively and promptly by the spiritual counselor alone.

- Remember that the "litmus test" of care coordination rests on the quality of the clinical documentation completed by all team members. Review one of your patient's clinical records and ask yourself the following:

"If I was unable to give a verbal report/update on this patient, would a peer be able to pick up and provide the same level of care and know (from the documentation) the current orders, including specific medications and other details that contribute to effective hospice care?"

## 8. QUALITY METRICS

- Are the patient's pain and other symptoms managed adequately?
- Is the patient's anxiety managed adequately?
- Is the patient's functional ability/status clearly documented?
- What is the condition of the patient's skin?
- Has the interdisciplinary POC been updated as changes occur and by all interdisciplinary group members?
- Are interventions providing comfort and maintaining dignity?

# BEDBOUND, COMA, AND SKIN CARE

## 1. GENERAL CONSIDERATIONS

Many hospice patients spend their last days in bed, depending on their diagnosis and health history. Although bedbound status is not a diagnosis, it is an important factor that affects all body systems and results in many teaching and guidance implications for family members and other caregivers.

- A coma is an outcome that can be a complication of many diagnoses. No matter the cause, management of the patient for comfort and dignity is the same.

- Interruption of skin integrity is a complication of many diagnoses. Again, no matter the cause, management of the patient for comfort and dignity is the same.

- Caregivers and family members are a vital element of effective patient care and safety in their own home setting.

## 2. ELIGIBILITY CONSIDERATIONS

Coma (any etiology):

- Comatose patients with any three of the following on day three of a coma:
  - Abnormal brain stem response
  - Absent verbal response
  - Absent withdrawal response to pain
  - Serum creatinine > 1.5 mg/dl
- Documentation of medical complications, in the context of progressive clinical decline within the previous 12 months, which supports a terminal prognosis:
  - Aspiration pneumonia
  - Upper urinary tract infection (pyelonephritis)
  - Sepsis

- Refractory stage 3–4 pressure ulcers
- Fever recurrent after antibiotics (CMS, 2015)

When addressing bedbound, coma, and skin care, refer to your MAC or other regulatory bodies for up-to-date and specific guidance.

## 3. POTENTIAL DIAGNOSES ICD-10-CM DIAGNOSTIC CODING

*The International Statistical Classification of Diseases and Related Health Problems* 10th Revision (ICD-10-CM) is a coding of diseases and signs, symptoms, abnormal findings, complaints, social circumstances, and external causes of injury or diseases, as classified by the WHO. The following diagnoses and codes are some of the most common conditions seen in this diagnosis. There are specific coding rules and conventions in the official coding manual that must be followed, and these rules may not be included in online websites or EMR software. Consult with a credentialed coder for any questions related to accurate coding.

### Bedbound

Bedbound codes should be used in conjunction with patient primary terminal diagnosis and other diagnoses that contribute to the terminal prognosis.

Z74.01 Bed confinement status

Z74.01 Bedridden

Z74.01 Status (post) bed confinement

### Pressure Ulcers

Codes for pressure ulcers are in Category L89 in the ICD-10-CM and are combination codes that identify the site, stage, and (in most cases) laterality of the ulcer. Possible stages are 1–4 and unstagable.

- **Stage 1**—Skin changes limited to persistent, focal, nonblanchable erythema.
- **Stage 2**—An abrasion, blister, and partial thickness skin loss involving the dermis and epidermis.

- **Stage 3**—Full thickness skin loss with exposed adipose tissue.
- **Stage 4**—Necrosis of soft tissues exposing the underlying muscle, tendon, or bone.
- **Unstagable**—Based on clinical documentation, the stage cannot be determined clinically (for example, the wound is covered with eschar) or for ulcers documented as deep tissue injury without evidence of trauma.

Codes for nonpressure chronic ulcers are in Category L97 and L98 and have an instructional note to code first any associated underlying condition.

## 4. SAFETY CONSIDERATIONS

- Infection control and prevention/standard precautions (that is, disposal of soiled dressings)
- Side rail use and positioning
- Comprehensive skin care and assessment
- Proper positioning and frequent position changes (for physical safety and skin care)
- Nightlight
- Removal of scatter rugs
- Tub rail, grab bars for bathroom safety
- Smoking and oxygen safety
- Wheelchair/fall precautions
- Home medical equipment safety, including oxygen
- Supportive nonskid shoes and caution on slippery walking surfaces
- Smoke detector and fire evacuation plan
- Supervised care and medication regimen
- Assistance with transfers and ambulation
- Others, based on the patient's unique condition and environment

## 5. SKILLS AND SERVICES IDENTIFIED

## Registered Nurse

Various scales assess patient function, but the two scales that are used most commonly by hospice and palliative care professionals are the Palliative Performance Scale (PPS) and the Karnofsky Performance Scale (KPS).

*The Palliative Performance Scale (PPS)* is a tool that hospice and palliative care professionals use to measure progressive patient decline. The scale has five functional dimensions:

- Ambulation
- Activity level and evidence of disease
- Self-care
- Oral intake
- Level of consciousness

There are 11 defined levels of scoring, from 0% to 100%, in 10% increments on the tool. Every decrease in 10% marks a significant decrease in physical function. Determining the patient's PPS score serves as a way for the IDG to determine the patient's functional status. It is important that clinicians be trained to administer the scale and follow the scale instructions to ensure an accurate assessment (Anderson et al., 1995).

*The Karnofsky Performance Scale (KPS)* is a tool that measures the ability of a patient to perform ADLs and can be used for prognostic purposes. The KPS scores range from 0 to 10, and the higher the score, the better a patient can carry out daily activities (Schag et al., 1984).

### *Comfort and Symptom Management*
**Assess**

- Completion of initial and comprehensive assessment of all systems of patient admitted to hospice for _____ (specify problem necessitating care)
- Assessment of vital signs every visit

- Assessment of patient, family, and caregiver wishes and expectations regarding care
- Assessment of patient, family, and caregiver resources available for care
- Assessment of pain and other symptoms, including site, duration, and characteristics; evaluation of pain management's effectiveness; and identification of the need for change, addition, or another plan or dose adjustment

## Teach Patient and Family/Caregiver

- Presentation of hospice philosophy and services
- Explanation of patient rights and responsibilities
- Teaching physical care of patient
- Teaching about specific disease and management at end of life
- Teaching new pain and symptom control medication regimen
- Teaching symptom control and relief measures
- Teaching care of weak, terminally ill patient
- Instructing in pain control measures and medications
- Teaching about realistic expectations of the disease process
- Teaching care of the dying and identification of signs/symptoms of impending death

## Provide Care/Case Management

- Comprehensive care coordination with all members of the IDG and other healthcare providers
- Care plan oversight
- Skilled assessment and support of the patient, family, and caregiver's coping skills
- Medication management
- Home medical equipment as indicated
- Interventions of symptoms directed toward comfort and palliation

- Comfort measures of backrub and hand or other therapeutic massage
- Presence and support
- Volunteer support to patient and family per their request
- Other interventions, based on patient/family needs

## Safety and Mobility Considerations

- Caregiver provided with home safety information and instruction related to _____
- Teaching family regarding safety and observation of patient in home
- Teaching family regarding energy conservation techniques
- Teaching safe oral intake (especially liquids)
- Monitoring for choking/aspiration if oral intake is possible
- Teaching caregiver safe and effective suctioning of patient secretions
- Teaching caregiver/family safety related to bed mobility and transfers
- Other interventions, based on patient/family needs

## Emotional/Spiritual Considerations

- Psychosocial assessment of patient and family regarding disease and prognosis (may be completed by the RN or the hospice social worker)
- Providing emotional support to patient and family with _____, and illness of a terminal nature
- Assessment of mental status and sleep disturbance changes
- Assessment for signs/symptoms of depression
- Spiritual counseling/support offered to patients and caregiver who verbalize emotional or spiritual pain and turmoil
- Support to patient and family/caregivers
- Other interventions, based on patient/family needs

### Skin Considerations

**Assess**

- Assessment and observation of skin integrity and patient's physical status
- Observation and assessment/evaluation of any wound and surrounding skin
- Evaluation of patient's need for equipment/supplies to decrease pressure; alternating pressure mattress, gel foam seat cushion, and heel and elbow protectors
- Observation and assessment of areas for possible breakdown, including bony prominences and other pressure-prone areas

**Teach Patient and Family/Caregiver**

- Skin care related to patient's needs, including the need for frequent position changes, appropriate pressure pads and mattresses, effective use of turn/pull sheet to avoid friction, skin tears and burns, and the prevention of breakdown
- Proper body alignment and positioning in bed to prevent skin tears from shearing skin

**Provide Care**

- Palliative wound care that focuses on relieving suffering and improving the patient's quality of life when their wound no longer responds to, or the patient can no longer tolerate, curative treatment; it concentrates on symptom management, addressing the problems of infection, pain, wound odor, exudate, and decreased self-confidence in end-of-life care (Wound Source, 2017)
- Pressure ulcer care as indicated
  - Changing of dressing at wound site using aseptic technique of _____ (define ordered care)
  - Culturing of wound and urine and sending to lab (per physician order)

- Consideration of RN enterostomal therapist to visit patient and evaluate wound for specific palliative care needs
- Other interventions, based on patient/family needs

## Elimination Considerations

- Assessing bowel regimen and implementing program as needed
- Monitoring bowel patterns, including frequency of bowel movements, and evaluating bowel regimen (for example, stool softeners, laxatives, and dietary changes)
- Checking for and removing impaction per physician orders
- Implementing bladder training program
- Teaching caregiver daily catheter care and equipment care and signs and symptoms that necessitate calling the hospice
- Changing catheter (specify type, size, and frequency) as indicated
- Assessing amount and frequency of urinary output
- Other interventions, based on patient/family needs

## Hydration/Nutrition

- Assessing and monitoring hydration/nutrition status
- Providing diet counseling for patient with cachexia
- Teaching family/caregivers proper care of the feeding tube
- Supporting nutrition/hydration by offering patient's choice of favorite or desired foods or liquids
- Maintaining nutrition/hydration by offering patient high-protein diet and food of choice as tolerated
- Teaching patient and family to expect decreased nutritional and fluid intake as disease progresses
- Monitoring and recording weights as ordered
- Other interventions, based on patient/family needs

## Therapeutic/Medication Regimens

- Completing an assessment and reconciliation of all patient prescriptions and over-the-counter drugs, herbal remedies, and other alternative treatments that could affect drug therapy, including, but not limited to, identification of the following:
  - Effectiveness of drug therapy
  - Drug side effects
  - Actual or potential drug interactions
  - Duplicate drug therapy
  - Drug therapy currently associated with laboratory monitoring
- Instruction on all medications including schedule, functions of specific drugs, and their side effects/interactions
- Monitoring and assessing complications for new medication regimen
- Review of medication side effects and drug/drug, drug/food interactions
- Monitoring of patient's response to medications for pain and symptom control
- Monitoring adherence to medication regimen
- Assessment of patient's unique response to treatments or interventions, and report of changes or unfavorable responses or reactions to the physician
- Teaching new pain and symptom control medication regimen
- Teaching patient and family about new medications and side effects
- Obtaining venipuncture as ordered every _____ (order frequency)
- Teaching patient and caregiver use of PCA pump
- Assessment for electrolyte imbalance
- Nonpharmacological interventions such as progressive muscle relaxation, imagery, positive visualization, music, massage and touch, and humor therapy of patient's choice
- Other interventions, based on patient/family needs

## Other Considerations

- Assessment of disease progression
- Assistance to family in setting up patient-centered routine and stressing the importance of adhering to the routine once established
- Assessment of the patient's response to treatments and interventions and reporting to the physician any changes, unfavorable responses, or reactions
- Other interventions, based on patient/family needs

## Hospice Aide

- Effective and safe personal care
- Safe ADL assistance and support, ambulation, and transfers
- Observance of and report of any changes in patient condition
- Preparation or assistance with preparation of meals
- Homemaker services (as requested by family)
- Comfort care measures per patient needs and aide care plan
- Other duties as assigned and within the scope of practice

## Social Worker

- Completion of psychosocial assessment
- Support to patient and family/caregivers related to adjusting to the illness and its implications and the need for care
- Identification of optimal coping strategies
- Financial assessment and counseling regarding food acquisition and ability to prepare meals
- Interventions/support related to terminal illness and loss
- Emotional/spiritual support
- Facilitation of communication among patient, family, and hospice team
- Referrals/linkage to community services and resources as indicated

- Grief counseling and intervention/support related to illness/loss
- Identification of any illness-related psychiatric condition necessitating care
- Assistance with funeral and burial planning

## Volunteer(s)

- Support, friendship, companionship, and presence
- Comfort and dignity for patient and family
- Assistance with errands and transportation
- Other services based on interdisciplinary group recommendations and patient/caregiver needs

## Spiritual Counselor

- Spiritual assessment and care
- Counseling, interventions, and support related to life's meaning (consistent with patient's beliefs)
- Prayer with or for the patient's family using prayers familiar to patient's religious background (per their wishes)
- Support, listening, and presence
- Participation in sacred or spiritual rituals or practices
- Assistance with funeral planning
- Other supportive care, based on patient/family needs and belief systems

## Other Services

- Physical therapy, occupational therapy, and speech therapy as directed by a physician
- Nonpharmacological interventions such as progressive muscle relaxation, imagery, positive visualization, music, massage and touch, pet therapy (including patient's pets if available), and humor therapy of patient's choice

- Plans to engage patient and support comfort, quality, enjoyment, and dignity
- Evaluation and interventions based on patient's and caregiver's unique wishes and needs that support care, comfort, and death in the setting of the patient's choice when possible

## 6. PATIENT, FAMILY, AND CAREGIVER EDUCATIONAL NEEDS

Educational needs are the care regimens that contribute to safe and effective care at home between the hospice team's visits. These include the following:

- The basic tenets of hospice and the availability of support 24 hours a day, 7 days a week
- Home safety assessment and counseling
- Safe and proper body mechanics to promote patient comfort and prevent caregiver safety problems
- Support groups available to the patient's family, such as caregiver support groups
- Skin care regimens
- Catheter and wound care programs
- Effective personal hygiene habits
- Home exercise program, including range of motion
- Safety measures in the home when the patient is immobilized
- Infection control and prevention
- Medication regimen and the medications' relationships to each other
- Importance of medical follow-up
- When to call the hospice
- Anticipated disease progression
- Other information based on the patient's/family's unique needs

## 7. TIPS FOR QUALITY, SAFETY, ELIGIBILITY, AND REIMBURSEMENT

- The Medicare Hospice Benefit does not require that the patient be homebound or have identified skilled needs, but care must be medically necessary to qualify for Medicare reimbursement.

- Unless the patient has a hospice benefit, some insurers will not pay for a skilled nurse visit that is made at death if the patient is dead when the nurse arrives at the home.

- Should the patient's status deteriorate and increased personal care be needed, obtain a verbal order for the increased service, noting frequency and estimating the duration.

- Obtain a verbal order for all medication and skilled treatment changes (for example, antibiotic therapy), and document these in the clinical record.

- Document the symptoms and clinical assessment findings that support the terminal prognosis.

  - Patient changes, symptoms, and clinical information identified from visits and team meetings that support hospice care and limited life expectancy

    - Mentation, behavioral, and cognitive changes

    - Dysphagia, weight loss, dyspnea, infection, sepsis, and new or changed medications

    - Skin changes (for example, inflamed, painful, weeping skin site[s]) and reddened bony prominences

    - Dehydration

    - Patient change and decline

    - Pain, other symptoms not controlled

    - Status after acute episode of _____ (specify)

    - Positive urine, sputum culture; patient started

    - Febrile at _____, pulse change at _____, irregularly irregular

    - Medication adjustments

- Nutrition, hydration, or elimination concerns (for example, decreased intake, fecal impaction)
- Any variances to expected outcomes
- Inability to perform ADLs, personal care
- Frequent communication required with physician regarding _____ (specify)
- Clear support of the rationale that supports/explains the progression of the illness from the chronic to the terminal stages
- Coordination of services and consultations with other members of the IDG

- Document all IDG meetings and communications in the POC and in the progress notes of the clinical record.

- Document coordination of services or consultation providers, such as skilled nursing facility or nursing home staff, inpatient team members, and hired caregivers.

- Document what the patient looks like (frail, pale, poor intake, shortness of breath, inability to do ADLs, and so on).

- Ensure that all team members have provided input into the patient's POC and documented their interventions and goals.

- Remember that the clinical documentation is vital to measuring compliance for quality and reimbursement purposes. Care coordination, timely verbal and initial physician orders, and assessment and addressing of spiritual and psychosocial needs should be clearly documented in the patient's clinical record.

- Make sure the documentation maintains that all hospice care supports comfort and dignity while meeting patient/family needs.

- Ensure that all team members, including clinicians and social workers, assess, identify, and "hear" spiritual needs that the patient/family want to be addressed. These spiritual issues are important to the provision of quality hospice care and cannot be addressed effectively and promptly by the spiritual counselor alone.

- Remember that the "litmus test" of care coordination rests on the quality of the clinical documentation completed by all team members. Review one of your patient's clinical records and ask yourself the following:

  "If I was unable to give a verbal report/update on this patient, would a peer be able to pick up and provide the same level of care and know (from the documentation) the current orders, including specific medications and other details that contribute to effective hospice care?"

## 8. QUALITY METRICS

- Are patient's pain and other symptoms managed adequately?
- Is patient's anxiety managed adequately?
- Is the patient's functional ability/status clearly documented?
- What is the condition of the patient's skin?
- Has the interdisciplinary POC been updated as changes occur and by all interdisciplinary group members?
- Are interventions providing comfort and maintaining dignity?

# CANCER

## 1. GENERAL CONSIDERATIONS

The Medicare Hospice Benefit was created in 1983 to care for individuals at the end of life. At that time, most individuals admitted to hospice had a diagnosis of cancer.

## 2. ELIGIBILITY CONSIDERATIONS

Patient eligibility for hospice is determined by the hospice physician in consultation with the referring and/or patient's attending physician. Per MAC hospice LCDs, cancer with distant metastases at presentation or progression from an earlier stage of disease to metastatic disease is eligibility evidence for hospice care with either:

- A continued decline despite therapy
- A patient declining further disease-directed therapy

A patient with a cancer diagnosis should also meet a MAC's "Decline in Clinical Status Guidelines." The decline LCDs state:

> "Patients will be considered to have a life expectancy of six months or less if there is documented evidence of decline in clinical status based on the guidelines listed. Since determination of decline presumes assessment of the patient's status over time, it is essential that both baseline and follow-up determinations be reported where appropriate. Baseline data may be established on admission to hospice or by using existing information from records. These changes in clinical variables apply to patients whose decline is not considered to be reversible" (CGS, 2015).

Progression of disease is characterized by worsening clinical status, symptoms, signs and laboratory results, and functional status (functional assessment score).

> **NOTE** Certain cancers with poor prognoses (for example, small cell lung cancer, brain cancer, and pancreatic cancer) may be hospice-eligible without fulfilling the other criteria in this section.

When addressing cancer, refer to your MAC or other regulatory bodies for up-to-date and specific guidance.

## 3. POTENTIAL DIAGNOSES ICD-10-CM DIAGNOSTIC CODING

The *International Statistical Classification of Diseases and Related Health Problems* 10th Revision (ICD-10-CM) is a coding of diseases and signs, symptoms, abnormal findings, complaints, social circumstances, and external causes of injury or diseases, as classified by the WHO. There are specific coding rules and conventions in the official coding manual that must be followed; these rules may not be included in online websites or EMR software. Consult with a credentialed coder for any questions related to accurate coding.

> ICD-10-CM Chapter II contains cancer diagnoses codes. Neoplasms IC00–D48
>
> C00–C14 Malignant neoplasms, lip, oral cavity, and pharynx
>
> C15–C26 Malignant neoplasms, digestive organs
>
> C30–C39 Malignant neoplasms, respiratory system, and intrathoracic organs
>
> C40–C41 Malignant neoplasms, bone, and articular cartilage
>
> C43–C44 Malignant neoplasms, skin
>
> C45–C49 Malignant neoplasms, connective and soft tissue
>
> C50–C58 Malignant neoplasms, breast and female genital organs
>
> C60–C63 Malignant neoplasms of male genital organs
>
> C64–C68 Malignant neoplasms, urinary organs

C69–C72 Malignant neoplasms, eye, brain, and central nervous system

C73–C75 Malignant neoplasms, endocrine glands and related structures

C76–C80 Malignant neoplasms, secondary and ill-defined

C81–C96 Malignant neoplasms, stated or presumed to be primary, of lymphoid, hematopoietic, and related tissue

C97 Malignant neoplasms of independent (primary) multiple sites

D00–D09 In situ neoplasms

D10–D36 Benign neoplasms

D37–D48 Neoplasms of uncertain or unknown behavior

## 4. SAFETY CONSIDERATIONS

- Infection control and prevention/standard precautions
- Supervised medication administration
- Multiple medications safety (side effects, interactions, storage)
- Home medical equipment safety, including oxygen
- Nightlight
- Removal of scatter rugs
- Tub rail, grab bars for bathroom safety
- Supportive and nonskid shoes
- Smoking and oxygen safety
- Handrail on stairs
- Fall precautions
- Protective skin measures
- Use of handrails
- Smoke detector and fire evacuation plan
- Assistance with ambulation
- Supervised care and medication regimen
- Others, based on the patient's unique condition and environment

## 5. SKILLS AND SERVICES IDENTIFIED

## Registered Nurse

### Assess

Pain can be the primary symptom with a cancer diagnosis, and pain is whatever the patient says it is. Assessment using a designated pain measurement scale is necessary to develop a pain management plan. Common assessment scales used in hospice and palliative care are:

- 0–10 pain assessment scale—The patient is asked to rate his or her pain intensity and severity on a scale of 0–10.

- Wong-Baker FACES pain assessment scale—The patient is asked to rate his or her pain intensity and severity by pointing to a face that characterizes the pain (Wong-Baker Faces Foundation, 2016).

- A comprehensive assessment of the patient's pain should be based on accepted clinical standards of practice and include:

  - History of pain and its treatment (including nonpharmacological and pharmacological treatment)

  - Characteristics of pain, such as:

    - Intensity of pain (for example, as measured on a standardized pain scale)

    - Descriptors of pain (for example, burning, stabbing, tingling, aching)

    - Pattern of pain (for example, constant or intermittent)

    - Location and radiation of pain

    - Frequency, timing, and duration of pain

    - Impact of pain on quality of life (for example, on sleeping, functioning, appetite, and mood)

    - Factors such as activities, care, or treatment that precipitate or exacerbate pain

    - Strategies and factors that reduce pain

    - Additional symptoms associated with pain, including nausea and anxiety

- Physical examination (may include the pain site, the nervous system, mobility and function, and physical, psychological, and cognitive status)
- Current medical conditions and medications
- The patient's/family's goals for pain management and their satisfaction with the current level of pain control
- Comprehensive assessment of the cardiac, respiratory, and integumentary systems for a patient with cancer to determine related effects of the disease process and side effects of medication

## Comfort and Symptom Management

### Assess

- Completion of initial and comprehensive assessment of all systems of patient admitted to hospice for _____ (specify problem necessitating care)
- Assessment of vital signs every visit
- Assessment of patient, family, and caregiver wishes and expectations regarding care
- Assessment of patient, family, and caregiver resources available for care
- Assessment of pain and other symptoms, including site, duration, characteristics; evaluation of the pain management's effectiveness; identification of need for change, addition, or other plan or dose adjustment

### Teach Patient and Family/Caregiver

- Presentation of hospice philosophy and services
- Explanation of patient rights and responsibilities
- Teaching physical care of patient
- Teaching about specific disease and management at end of life

- Teaching new pain and symptom control medication regimen
- Teaching symptom control and relief measures
- Teaching care of weak, terminally ill patient
- Instruction in pain control measures and medications
- Teaching about realistic expectations of disease process
- Teaching care of the dying and identification of signs/symptoms of impending death

**Provide Care/Case Management**

- Comprehensive care coordination with all members of the IDG and other healthcare providers
- Care plan oversight
- Skilled assessment and support of the patient, family, and caregiver's coping skills
- Medication management
- Home medical equipment as indicated
- Interventions of symptoms directed toward comfort and palliation
- Comfort measures of backrub and hand or other therapeutic massage
- Presence and support
- Volunteer support to patient and family per their request
- Other interventions, based on patient/family needs

*Safety and Mobility Considerations*

- Providing caregiver with home safety information and instruction related to _____
- Teaching family regarding safety of patient in home
- Teaching family regarding energy conservation techniques
- Teaching safe oral intake (especially liquids)
- Monitoring for choking/aspiration if oral intake is possible

- Teaching caregiver safe and effective suctioning of patient secretions
- Teaching caregiver/family safety related to bed mobility and transfers
- Other interventions, based on patient/family needs

### Emotional/Spiritual Considerations

- Psychosocial assessment of patient and family regarding disease and prognosis (may be completed by the RN or the hospice social worker)
- Emotional support to patient and family with _____, and illness of a terminal nature
- Assessment of mental status and sleep disturbance changes
- Assessment for signs/symptoms of depression
- Spiritual counseling/support to patients and caregivers who verbalize emotional or spiritual pain and turmoil
- Support to patient and family/caregivers
- Other interventions, based on patient/family needs

### Skin Considerations

**Assess**

- Assessment and observation of skin integrity and patient's physical status
- Observation and assessment/evaluation of any wound and surrounding skin
- Evaluation of patient's need for equipment/supplies to decrease pressure; alternating pressure mattress, gel foam seat cushion, and heel and elbow protectors
- Observation and assessment of areas for possible breakdown, including bony prominences and other pressure-prone areas

**Teach Patient and Family/Caregiver**

- Skin care related to patient's needs, including the need for frequent position changes, appropriate pressure pads and mattresses, effective use of turn/pull sheet to avoid friction, skin tears and burns, and the prevention of breakdown
- Proper body alignment and positioning in bed to prevent skin tears from shearing skin

**Provide Care**

- Palliative wound care that focuses on relieving suffering and improving the patient's quality of life when the wound no longer responds to, or the patient can no longer tolerate, curative treatment; palliative wound care concentrates on symptom management, addressing the problems of infection, pain, wound odor, exudate, and decreased self-confidence in end-of-life care (Wound Source, 2017)
- Pressure ulcer care as indicated
  - Change dressing at wound site using aseptic technique of _____ (define ordered care)
  - Culturing of wound and urine and sending to lab (per physician order)
  - Consideration of RN enterostomal therapist to visit patient and evaluate wound for specific palliative care needs
- Other interventions, based on patient/family needs

### Elimination Considerations

- Assessment of bowel regimen, and implementation of program as needed
- Monitoring of bowel patterns, including frequency of bowel movements, and evaluating bowel regimen (for example, stool softeners, laxatives, and dietary changes)
- Checking for and removing impaction per physician orders
- Implementing bladder training program

- Teaching caregiver daily catheter care and equipment care and signs and symptoms that necessitate calling the hospice
- Changing catheter (specify type, size, and frequency) as indicated
- Assessing amount and frequency of urinary output
- Other interventions, based on patient/family needs

## Hydration/Nutrition

- Assessing and monitoring hydration/nutrition status
- Providing diet counseling for patient with cachexia
- Teaching family/caregivers proper care of the feeding tube
- Supporting nutrition/hydration by offering patient's choice of favorite or desired foods or liquids
- Maintaining nutrition/hydration by offering patient high-protein diet and food of choice as tolerated
- Teaching patient and family to expect decreased nutritional and fluid intake as disease progresses
- Monitoring and recording weights as ordered
- Other interventions, based on patient/family needs

## Therapeutic/Medication Regimens

- Completion of an assessment and reconciliation of all patient prescriptions and over-the-counter drugs, herbal remedies, and other alternative treatments that could affect drug therapy, including, but not limited to, identification of the following:
  - Effectiveness of drug therapy
  - Drug side effects
  - Actual or potential drug interactions
  - Duplicate drug therapy
  - Drug therapy currently associated with laboratory monitoring
- Instruction on all medications including schedule, functions of specific drugs, and their side effects/interactions

- Monitoring and assessing complications for new medication regimen
- Managing medications-related drug/drug, drug/food side effects
- Monitoring patient's response to medications for pain and symptom control
- Monitoring adherence to medication regimen
- Assessing the patient's unique response to treatments or interventions, and reporting changes or unfavorable responses or reactions to the physician
- Teaching new pain and symptom control medication regimen
- Teaching patient and family about new medications and side effects
- Obtaining venipuncture as ordered every _____ (order frequency)
- Teaching patient and caregiver use of PCA pump
- Assessment for electrolyte imbalance
- Nonpharmacological interventions such as progressive muscle relaxation, imagery, positive visualization, music, massage and touch, and humor therapy of patient's choice
- Other interventions, based on patient/family needs

## Other Considerations

- Assessing disease progression
- Assisting family in setting up patient-centered routine and stressing the importance of adhering to the routine once established
- Assessing the patient's response to treatments and interventions and reporting to the physician any changes, unfavorable responses, or reactions
- Other interventions, based on patient/family needs

### Hospice Aide

- Effective and safe personal care
- Assurance of safe ADL assistance and support, ambulation, and transfers

- Observation and reporting of any changes in patient condition
- Preparation or assistance with preparation of meals
- Homemaker services (as requested by family)
- Comfort care measures per patient needs and aide care plan
- Other duties as assigned and within the scope of practice

**Social Worker**

- Completion of psychosocial assessment
- Support to patient and families/caregivers related to adjusting to the illness and its implications and the need for care
- Identification of optimal coping strategies
- Financial assessment and counseling regarding food acquisition and ability to prepare meals
- Interventions/support related to terminal illness and loss
- Emotional/spiritual support
- Facilitation of communication among patient, family, and hospice team
- Referrals/linkage to community services and resources as indicated
- Grief counseling and intervention/support related to illness/loss
- Identification of any illness-related psychiatric condition necessitating care
- Assistance with funeral and burial planning

**Volunteer(s)**

- Support, friendship, companionship, and presence
- Comfort and dignity for patient and family
- Assistance with errands and transportation
- Other services based on interdisciplinary group recommendations and patient/caregiver needs

**Spiritual Counselor**

- Spiritual assessment and care
- Counseling, interventions, and support related to life's meaning (consistent with patient's beliefs)
- Prayer with or for the patient's family using prayers familiar to patient's religious background (per their wishes)
- Support, listening, and presence
- Participation in sacred or spiritual rituals or practices
- Assistance with funeral planning
- Other supportive care, based on patient/family needs and belief systems

### Other Services

- Physical therapy, occupational therapy, and speech therapy as directed by a physician
- Nonpharmacological interventions such as progressive muscle relaxation, imagery, positive visualization, music, massage and touch, pet therapy (including patient's pets if available), and humor therapy of patient's choice
- Plans to engage patient and support comfort, quality, enjoyment, and dignity
- Evaluation and interventions based on patient's and caregiver's unique wishes and needs that support care, comfort, and death in the setting of the patient's choice when possible

## 6. PATIENT, FAMILY, AND CAREGIVER EDUCATIONAL NEEDS

Educational needs are the care regimens that contribute to safe and effective care at home between the hospice team's visits. These include the following:

- The basic tenets of hospice and the availability of support 24 hours a day, 7 days a week

- Home safety assessment and counseling
- Safe and proper body mechanics to promote patient comfort and prevent caregiver safety problems
- Support groups available to the patient's family, such as caregiver support groups
- Skin care regimens
- Catheter and wound care programs
- Effective personal hygiene habits
- Home exercise program, including range of motion
- Safety measures in the home when the patient is immobilized
- Infection control and prevention
- Medication regimen and the medications' relationships to each other
- Importance of medical follow-up
- When to call the hospice
- Anticipated disease progression
- Other information based on the patient's/family's unique needs

## 7. TIPS FOR QUALITY, SAFETY, ELIGIBILITY, AND REIMBURSEMENT

- Know that the Medicare Hospice Benefit does not require that the patient be homebound or have identified skilled needs, but care must be medically necessary to qualify for Medicare reimbursement.
- Recognize that, unless the patient has a hospice benefit, some insurers will not pay for a skilled nurse visit that is made at death if the patient is dead when the nurse arrives at the home.
- Should the patient's status deteriorate and increased personal care be needed, obtain a verbal order for the increased service, noting the frequency and estimating the duration.

- Obtain a verbal order for all medication and skilled treatment changes (for example, antibiotic therapy), and document these in the clinical record.
- Document the symptoms and clinical assessment findings that support the terminal prognosis.
  - Patient changes, symptoms, and clinical information identified from visits and team meetings that support hospice care and limited life expectancy
    - Mentation, behavioral, and cognitive changes
    - Dysphagia, weight loss, dyspnea, infection, sepsis, and new or changed medications
    - Skin changes (for example, inflamed, painful, weeping skin site[s]) and reddened bony prominences
    - Dehydration
    - Patient change and decline
    - Pain, other symptoms not controlled
    - Status after acute episode of _____ (specify)
    - Positive urine, sputum culture; patient started
    - Febrile at _____, pulse change at _____, irregularly irregular
    - Medication adjustments
    - Nutrition, hydration, or elimination concerns (for example, decreased intake, fecal impaction)
    - Any variances to expected outcomes
    - Inability to perform ADLs, personal care
    - Frequent communication required with physician regarding _____ (specify)
  - Clear support of the rationale that supports/explains the progression of the illness from the chronic to the terminal stages
  - Coordination of services and consultations with other members of the IDG

- Document all IDG meetings and communications in the POC and in the progress notes of the clinical record.

- Document coordination of services or consultation providers, such as skilled nursing facility or nursing home staff, inpatient team members, and hired caregivers.

- Document what the patient looks like (frail, pale, poor intake, shortness of breath, inability to do ADLs, and so on).

- Ensure that all team members have provided input into the patient's POC and documented their interventions and goals.

- Remember that the clinical documentation is vital to measuring compliance for quality and reimbursement purposes. Care coordination, timely verbal and initial physician orders, and assessment and addressing of spiritual and psychosocial needs should be clearly documented in the patient's clinical record.

- Make sure that the documentation maintains that all hospice care supports comfort and dignity while meeting patient/family needs.

- Ensure that all team members, including clinicians and social workers, assess, identify, and "hear" spiritual needs that the patient/family want to be addressed. These spiritual issues are important to the provision of quality hospice care and cannot be addressed effectively and promptly by the spiritual counselor alone.

- Remember that the "litmus test" of care coordination rests on the quality of the clinical documentation completed by all team members. Review one of your patient's clinical records and ask yourself the following:

  "If I was unable to give a verbal report/update on this patient, would a peer be able to pick up and provide the same level of care and know (from the documentation) the current orders, including specific medications and other details that contribute to effective hospice care?"

## 8. QUALITY METRICS

- Are the patient's pain and other symptoms managed adequately?
- Is the patient's anxiety managed adequately?
- Is the patient's functional ability/status clearly documented?
- What is the condition of the patient's skin?
- Has the interdisciplinary POC been updated as changes occur and by all interdisciplinary group members?
- Are interventions providing comfort and maintaining dignity?

# CARDIAC AND CEREBROVASCULAR ACCIDENT (STROKE) CARE

## 1. GENERAL CONSIDERATIONS

Patients and families may be referred to hospice for progressive and cardiac disease that can include cardiac myopathies, severe congestive heart failure, angina, post myocardial infarctions, and many other cardiac problems. These patients and their families have usually had a long history of aggressive treatment directed toward the cardiac disease. Supportive and skillful care is directed toward comfort and symptomatic relief of chest pain, shortness of breath, and other problems.

## 2. ELIGIBILITY CONSIDERATIONS

Patient eligibility for hospice is determined by the hospice physician in consultation with the referring and/or the patient's attending physician. The Medicare Administrative Contractor (MAC) hospice local coverage determinations (LCDs) for cardiac disease should be used by the physician and hospice team when making the eligibility determination.

### End-Stage Cardiac Disease

Per MAC, hospice LCDs patients are considered to be in the terminal stage of heart disease if they meet the following criteria:

- At the time of initial certification or recertification for hospice, the patient is or has been already optimally treated for heart disease or is not a candidate for a surgical procedure or has declined a procedure. (Optimally treated means that patients who are not on vasodilators have a medical reason for refusing these drugs, such as hypotension or renal disease.)

- The patient is classified as New York Heart Association (NYHA) Class IV and may have significant symptoms of heart failure or angina at rest. Significant congestive heart failure may be documented by an ejection fraction of ≤ 20%, but is not required if it is not already available.

- Documentation of the following factors support eligibility for hospice care:
  - Treatment-resistant symptomatic supraventricular or ventricular arrhythmias
  - History of cardiac arrest or resuscitation
  - History of unexplained syncope
  - Brain embolism of cardiac origin
  - Concomitant HIV disease (CGS, 2015)

## CVA (Stroke)

- Karnofsky Performance Scale (KPS) or Palliative Performance Scale (PPS) of 40% or less
- Inability to maintain hydration and caloric intake with one of the following:
  - Weight loss > 10% in the past 6 months or > 7.5% in the past 3 months
  - Serum albumin < 2.5 gm/dl
  - Current history of pulmonary aspiration not responsive to speech language pathology intervention
  - Sequential calorie counts documenting inadequate caloric/fluid intake
  - Dysphagia severe enough to prevent the patient from receiving food and fluids necessary to sustain life, in a patient who declines or does not receive artificial nutrition and hydration

When addressing CVA and stroke, refer to your MAC or other regulatory bodies for up-to-date and specific guidance.

## 3. POTENTIAL DIAGNOSES ICD-10-CM DIAGNOSTIC CODING

The *International Statistical Classification of Diseases and Related Health Problems* 10th Revision (ICD-10-CM) is a coding of diseases and signs, symptoms, abnormal findings, complaints, social circumstances and external causes of injury or diseases, as classified by the WHO. The following diagnoses and codes are some of the most common conditions seen in this diagnosis. There are specific coding rules and conventions in the official coding manual that must be followed, and these rules may not be included in online websites or EMR software. Consult with a credentialed coder for any questions related to accurate coding.

## Heart Failure

I50.1 Left ventricular failure

I50.20 Unspecified systolic heart failure

I50.21 Acute systolic heart failure

I50.22 Chronic systolic heart failure

I50.23 Acute on chronic systolic heart failure

I50.30 Unspecified diastolic heart failure

I50.31 Acute diastolic heart failure

I50.32 Chronic diastolic heart failure

I50.33 Acute on chronic diastolic heart failure

I50.30 Unspecified systolic and diastolic heart failure

I50.31 Acute systolic and diastolic heart failure

I50.32 Chronic systolic and diastolic heart failure

I50.33 Acute on chronic systolic and diastolic heart failure

I50.40 Unspecified systolic and diastolic heart failure

I50.41 Acute systolic and diastolic heart failure

I50.42 Chronic systolic and diastolic heart failure

I50.43 Acute on chronic systolic and diastolic heart failure

## CVA (Stroke)

I60–I62 Nontraumatic intracranial hemorrhage (that is spontaneous subarachnoid, intracerebral, or subdural hemorrhages)

I63 Cerebral infarctions (for example, due to a vessel thrombosis or embolus)

I65–I66 Occlusion and stenosis of cerebral or precerebral vessels without infarction

I67–I68 Other cerebrovascular diseases

I69 Sequelae of cerebrovascular disease (late effect)

## 4. SAFETY CONSIDERATIONS

- Infection control and prevention/standard precautions
- Supervised medication administration
- Multiple medications safety (side effects, interactions, storage)
- Smoking and oxygen safety
- Home medical equipment safety
- Nightlight
- Removal of scatter rugs
- Tub rail, grab bars for bathroom safety
- Supportive and nonskid shoes
- Handrails on stairs
- Fall precautions
- Protective skin measures
- Stairway precautions
- Smoke detector and fire evacuation plan
- Assistance with ambulation
- Supervised care and medication regimen
- Others, based on the patient's unique condition and environment

## 5. SKILLS AND SERVICES IDENTIFIED

## Registered Nurse

### Comfort and Symptom Management

**Assess**

- Completion of initial and comprehensive assessment of all systems of patient admitted to hospice for _____ (specify problem necessitating care)
- Assessment of vital signs every visit
- Assessment of heart rate, rhythm, and strength of heartbeat
- Assessment of lung sounds for congestion or other adventitious sounds
- Assessment for edema, including site and degree
- Assessment of dyspnea, including its effect on activity and quality of life
- Assessment of oxygen saturation and skin color
- Assessment for bruising and other complications related to anticoagulation therapy
- Assessment of fatigue level and its impact on ADLs
- Assessment for depression
- Assessment of mobility and appropriate use of assistive devices
- Assessment of patient, family, and caregiver wishes and expectations regarding care
- Assessment of patient, family, and caregiver resources available for care
- Assessment of pain and other symptoms, including site, duration, and characteristics; evaluation of the pain management's effectiveness; and identification of the need for change, addition, or another plan or dose adjustment

**Teach Patient and Family/Caregiver**

- Presentation of hospice philosophy and services
- Explanation of patient rights and responsibilities

- Teaching physical care of patient
- Teaching about specific disease and management at end of life
- Teach symptom control and relief measures
- Teaching care of weak, terminally ill patient
- Instruction in pain control measures and medications
- Teaching about realistic expectations of disease process
- Teaching care of the dying and identification of signs/symptoms of impending death

**Provide Care/Case Management**

- Comprehensive care coordination with all members of the IDG and other healthcare providers
- Care plan oversight
- Skilled assessment and support of the patient, family, and caregiver's coping skills
- Medication management
- Home medical equipment as indicated
- Interventions of symptoms directed toward comfort and palliation
- Comfort measures of backrub and hand or other therapeutic massage
- Presence and support
- Volunteer support to patient and family per their request
- Other interventions, based on patient/family needs

### Safety and Mobility Considerations

- Providing caregiver with home safety information and instruction related to _____
- Teaching family regarding safety of patient in home
- Teaching family regarding bleeding precautions for patients on anticoagulant therapy
- Teaching family regarding energy conservation techniques

- Teaching safe oral intake (especially liquids) for CVA patients
- Monitor for choking/aspiration in CVA patients
- Teaching caregiver safe and effective suctioning of patient secretions
- Teaching caregiver/family safety related to bed mobility and transfers
- Other interventions, based on patient/family needs

## Emotional/Spiritual Considerations

- Psychosocial assessment of patient and family regarding disease and prognosis (may be completed by the RN or the hospice social worker)
- Emotional support to patient and family with _____, and illness of a terminal nature
- Assessment of mental status and sleep disturbance changes
- Assessment of signs/symptoms of depression
- Spiritual counseling/support offered to patients and caregiver who verbalize emotional or spiritual pain and turmoil
- Support to patient and family/caregivers
- Other interventions, based on patient/family needs

## Skin Considerations

**Assess**

- Assessment and observation of skin integrity and patient's physical status
- Observation and assessment/evaluation of any wound and surrounding skin
- Evaluation of patient's need for equipment/supplies to decrease pressure; alternating pressure mattress, gel foam seat cushion, and heel and elbow protectors
- Observation and skilled assessment of areas for possible breakdown, including bony prominences and other pressure-prone areas

**Teach Patient and Family/Caregiver**

- Skin care related to patient's needs, including the need for frequent position changes, appropriate pressure pads and mattresses, effective use of turn/pull sheet to avoid friction, skin tears and burns, and the prevention of breakdown
- Proper body alignment and positioning in bed to prevent skin tears from shearing skin

**Provide Care**

- Palliative wound care that focuses on relieving suffering and improving the patient's quality of life when the wound no longer responds to, or the patient can no longer tolerate, curative treatment; palliative wound care concentrates on symptom management, addressing the problems of infection, pain, wound odor, exudate, and decreased self-confidence in end-of-life care (Wound Source, 2017)
- Pressure ulcer care as indicated
  - Changing dressing at wound site using aseptic technique of _____ (define ordered care)
  - Culturing wound and urine and sending to lab (per physician order)
  - Consideration of RN enterostomal therapist to visit patient and evaluate wound for specific palliative care needs
- Other interventions, based on patient/family needs

*Elimination Considerations*

- Assessing bowel regimen, and implementation of program as needed
- Monitoring of bowel patterns, including frequency of bowel movements, and evaluation of bowel regimen (for example, stool softeners, laxatives, and dietary changes)
- Checking for and removing impaction per physician orders
- Implementing bladder training program

- Teaching caregiver daily catheter care and equipment care and signs and symptoms that necessitate calling the hospice
- Changing catheter (specify type, size, and frequency) as indicated
- Assessing amount and frequency of urinary output
- Other interventions, based on patient/family needs

## *Hydration/Nutrition*

- Assessing and monitoring hydration/nutrition status
- Providing diet counseling for patient with cachexia
- Teaching family/caregivers proper care of the feeding tube
- Supporting nutrition/hydration by offering patient's choice of favorite or desired foods or liquids
- Maintaining nutrition/hydration by offering patient high-protein diet and food of choice as tolerated
- Teaching patient and family to expect decreased nutritional and fluid intake as disease progresses
- Monitoring and recording weights as ordered
- Other interventions, based on patient/family needs

## *Therapeutic/Medication Regimens*

- Completion of an assessment and reconciliation of all patient prescriptions and over-the-counter drugs, herbal remedies, and other alternative treatments that could affect drug therapy, including, but not limited to, identification of the following:
  - Effectiveness of drug therapy
  - Drug side effects
  - Actual or potential drug interactions
  - Duplicate drug therapy
  - Drug therapy currently associated with laboratory monitoring
- Instruction on all medications including schedule and functions of specific drugs and their side effects/interactions

- Monitoring and assessing complications for new medication regimen
- Managing medications related to drug/drug, drug/food side effects
- Monitoring patient's response to medications for pain and symptom control
- Monitoring adherence to medication regimen
- Assessing the patient's unique response to treatments or interventions, and reporting changes or unfavorable responses or reactions to the physician
- Teaching new pain and symptom control medication regimen
- Teaching patient and family about new medications and side effects
- Obtaining venipuncture as ordered every _____ (order frequency)
- Teaching patient and caregiver use of PCA pump
- Assessing electrolyte imbalance
- Nonpharmacological interventions such as progressive muscle relaxation, imagery, positive visualization, music, massage and touch, and humor therapy of patient's choice
- Other interventions, based on patient/family needs

### Other Considerations

- Assessing disease progression
- Assisting family in setting up patient-centered routine and stressing the importance of adhering to the routine once established
- Assessing the patient's response to treatments and interventions and reporting to the physician any changes, unfavorable responses, or reactions
- Other interventions, based on patient/family needs

### Hospice Aide

- Effective and safe personal care
- Assurance of safe ADL assistance and support, ambulation, and transfers

- Observance and report of any changes in patient condition
- Preparation or assistance with preparation of meals
- Homemaker services (as requested by family)
- Comfort care measures per patient needs and aide care plan
- Other duties as assigned and within the scope of practice

**Social Worker**

- Completion of psychosocial assessment
- Support to patient and family/caregivers related to adjusting to the illness and its implications and the need for care
- Identification of optimal coping strategies
- Financial assessment and counseling regarding food acquisition and ability to prepare meals
- Interventions/support related to terminal illness and loss
- Emotional/spiritual support
- Facilitation of communication among patient, family, and hospice team
- Referrals/linkage to community services and resources as indicated
- Grief counseling and intervention/support related to illness/loss
- Identification of any illness-related psychiatric condition necessitating care
- Assistance with funeral and burial planning

**Volunteer(s)**

- Support, friendship, companionship, and presence
- Comfort and dignity for patient and family
- Assistance with errands and transportation
- Other services based on interdisciplinary group recommendations and patient/caregiver needs

**Spiritual Counselor**

- Spiritual assessment and care
- Counseling, interventions, and support related to life's meaning (consistent with patient's beliefs)
- Prayer with or for the patient's family using prayers familiar to patient's religious background (per their wishes)
- Support, listening, and presence
- Participation in sacred or spiritual rituals or practices
- Assistance with funeral planning
- Other supportive care based on patient/family needs and belief systems

*Other Services*

- Physical therapy, occupational therapy, and speech therapy as directed by a physician
- Nonpharmacological interventions such as progressive muscle relaxation, imagery, positive visualization, music, massage and touch, pet therapy (including patient's pets if available), and humor therapy of patient's choice
- Plans to engage patient and support comfort, quality, enjoyment, and dignity
- Evaluation and interventions based on patient's and caregiver's unique wishes and needs that support care, comfort, and death in the setting of the patient's choice when possible

## 6. PATIENT, FAMILY, AND CAREGIVER EDUCATIONAL NEEDS

Educational needs are the care regimens that contribute to safe and effective care at home between the hospice team's visits. These include the following:

- The basic tenets of hospice and the availability of support 24 hours a day, 7 days a week

- Home safety assessment and counseling
- Safe and proper body mechanics to promote patient comfort and prevent caregiver safety problems
- Support groups available to the patient's family, such as caregiver support groups
- Skin care regimens
- Catheter and wound care programs
- Effective personal hygiene habits
- Home exercise program, including range of motion
- Safety measures in the home when the patient is immobilized
- Infection control and prevention
- Medication regimen and the medications' relationships to each other
- Importance of medical follow-up
- When to call the hospice
- Anticipated disease progression
- Other information based on the patient's/family's unique needs

## 7. TIPS FOR QUALITY, SAFETY, ELIGIBILITY, AND REIMBURSEMENT

- Know that the Medicare Hospice Benefit does not require that the patient be homebound or have identified skilled needs, but care must be medically necessary to qualify for Medicare reimbursement.
- Understand that unless the patient has a hospice benefit, some insurers will not pay for a skilled nurse visit that is made at death if the patient is dead when the nurse arrives at the home.
- Should the patient's status deteriorate and increased personal care be needed, obtain a verbal order for the increased service, noting frequency and estimating the duration.

- Obtain a verbal order for all medication and skilled treatment changes (for example, antibiotic therapy), and document these in the clinical record.
- Document the symptoms and clinical assessment findings that support the terminal prognosis.
  - Patient changes, symptoms, and clinical information identified from visits and team meetings that support hospice care and limited life expectancy
    - Mentation, behavioral, and cognitive changes
    - Dysphagia, weight loss, dyspnea, infection, sepsis, and new or changed medications
    - Skin changes (for example, inflamed, painful, weeping skin site[s]) and reddened bony prominences
    - Dehydration
    - Patient change and decline
    - Pain and other symptoms not controlled
    - Status after acute episode of _____ (specify)
    - Positive urine, sputum culture; patient started
    - Febrile at _____, pulse change at _____, irregularly irregular
    - Medication adjustments
    - Nutrition, hydration, or elimination concerns (for example, decreased intake, fecal impaction)
    - Any variances to expected outcomes
    - Inability to perform ADLs, personal care
    - Frequent communication required with physician regarding _____ (specify)
  - Clear support of the rationale that supports/explains the progression of the illness from the chronic to the terminal stages
  - Coordination of services and consultations with other members of the IDG

- Document all IDG meetings and communications in the POC and in the progress notes of the clinical record.

- Document coordination of services or consultation providers, such as skilled nursing facility or nursing home staff, inpatient team members, and hired caregivers.

- Document what the patient looks like (frail, pale, poor intake, shortness of breath, inability to do ADLs, and so on).

- Ensure that all team members have provided input into the patient's POC and documented their interventions and goals.

- Remember that the clinical documentation is vital to measuring compliance for quality and reimbursement purposes. Care coordination, timely verbal and initial physician orders, and assessment and addressing of spiritual and psychosocial needs should be clearly documented in the patient's clinical record.

- Make sure that the documentation maintains that all hospice care supports comfort and dignity while meeting patient/family needs.

- Ensure that all team members, including clinicians and social workers, assess, identify, and "hear" spiritual needs that the patient/family want to be addressed. These spiritual issues are important to the provision of quality hospice care and cannot be addressed effectively and promptly by the spiritual counselor alone.

- Remember that the "litmus test" of care coordination rests on the quality of the clinical documentation completed by all team members. Review one of your patient's clinical records and ask yourself the following:

  "If I was unable to give a verbal report/update on this patient, would a peer be able to pick up and provide the same level of care and know (from the documentation) the current orders, including specific medications and other details that contribute to effective hospice care?"

## 8. QUALITY METRICS

- Are the patient's pain and other symptoms managed adequately?
- Is the patient's anxiety managed adequately?
- Is the patient's functional ability/status clearly documented?
- What is the condition of the patient's skin?
- Has the interdisciplinary POC been updated as changes occur and by all interdisciplinary group members?
- Are interventions providing comfort and maintaining dignity?

# LIVER DISEASE CARE

## 1. GENERAL CONSIDERATIONS

End-stage liver disease (ESLD) is a leading cause of death in people between the ages of 25 and 64 years in the United States. Patients with ESLD require progressive medical support and manifest a range of complications and symptoms that have significant impact on both survival and quality of life (Cox-North, Doorenbos, Shannon, Scott, & Curtis, 2013).

## 2. ELIGIBILITY CONSIDERATIONS

Patients are considered to be in the terminal stage of liver disease if they meet the following criteria:

- Prothrombin time prolonged more than 5 seconds over control, or International Normalized Ratio (INR) > 1.5
- Serum albumin < 2.5 gm/dl
- End-stage liver disease is present, and the patient shows at least one of the following:
  - Ascites, refractory to treatment, or patient noncompliant
  - Spontaneous bacterial peritonitis
  - Hepatorenal syndrome (elevated creatinine and BUN with oliguria < 400 ml/day and urine sodium concentration < 10 mEq/l)
  - Hepatic encephalopathy, refractory to treatment, or patient noncompliant
  - Recurrent variceal bleeding, despite intensive therapy
- Documentation of the following factors, which support eligibility for hospice care:
  - Progressive malnutrition
  - Muscle wasting with reduced strength and endurance
  - Continued active alcoholism (> 80 gm ethanol/day)

- Hepatocellular carcinoma
- HBsAg (Hepatitis B) positivity
- Hepatitis C refractory to interferon treatment

Patients awaiting liver transplant who otherwise fit the preceding criteria may be certified for the Medicare Hospice Benefit, but if a donor organ is procured, the patient must be discharged from hospice (Palmetto GBA, 2017).

When addressing liver disease, refer to your MAC or other regulatory bodies for up-to-date and specific guidance.

## 3. POTENTIAL DIAGNOSES ICD-10-CM DIAGNOSTIC CODING

The *International Statistical Classification of Diseases and Related Health Problems* 10th Revision (ICD-10-CM) is a coding of diseases and signs, symptoms, abnormal findings, complaints, social circumstances, and external causes of injury or diseases, as classified by the WHO. There are specific coding rules and conventions in the official coding manual that must be followed, and these rules may not be included in online websites or EMR software. Consult with a credentialed coder for any questions related to accurate coding.

Liver disease codes are in ICD-10-CM Chapter XI, "Diseases of the Digestive System."

K00–K93 Diseases of the digestive system

K70–K77 Diseases of liver

K72 Hepatic failure, not elsewhere classified

## 4. SAFETY CONSIDERATIONS

- Infection control and prevention/standard precautions
- Supervised medication administration
- Multiple medication safety (side effects, interactions, storage)
- Home medical equipment safety, including oxygen

- Nightlight
- Removal of scatter rugs
- Tub rail, grab bars for bathroom safety
- Supportive and nonskid shoes
- Smoking with supervision only
- Handrail on stairs
- Fall precautions
- Protective skin measures
- Stairway precautions
- Smoke detector and fire evacuation plan
- Assistance with ambulation
- Supervised care and medication regimen
- Others, based on the patient's unique condition and environment

## 5. SKILLS AND SERVICES IDENTIFIED

### Registered Nurse

**Assess**

- Comprehensive assessment of gastrointestinal system, integumentary system, cardiopulmonary systems, and endocrine system. Signs and symptoms of liver failure include:
  - Fatigue
  - Anorexia
  - Malaise
  - Weight loss/gain
  - Fever
  - Pruritus
  - Right upper quadrant or other pain
  - Gastrointestinal bleeding
  - Mental state shows drowsiness and possibly confusion
  - Jaundice

- Abdominal distension and abdominal masses, including:
  - Possible massive ascites and anasarca due to fluid redistribution and hypoalbuminemia (a dehydrated patient may not show much ascites)
  - Hepatomegaly and splenomegaly, but not invariably
- Cerebral edema with increased intracranial pressure (ICP) may produce papilledema, hypertension, and bradycardia (Mayo Clinic, 2017a).

## Comfort and Symptom Management

### Assess

- Completion of initial and comprehensive assessment of all systems of patient admitted to hospice for _____ (specify problem necessitating care)
- Assessment of vital signs every visit
- Assessment of patient, family, and caregiver wishes and expectations regarding care
- Assessment of patient, family, and caregiver resources available for care
- Assessment of pain and other symptoms, including site, duration, and characteristics; evaluation of the pain management's effectiveness; and identification of the need for change, addition, or another plan or dose adjustment

### Teach Patient and Family/Caregiver

- Presentation of hospice philosophy and services
- Explanation of patient rights and responsibilities
- Teaching physical care of patient
- Teaching about specific disease and management at end of life
- Teaching new pain and symptom control medication regimen
- Teaching symptom control and relief measures
- Teaching care of weak, terminally ill patient

- Instruction in pain control measures and medications
- Teaching about realistic expectations of disease process
- Teaching care of the dying and identification of signs/symptoms of impending death

**Provide Care/Case Management**

- Comprehensive care coordination with all members of the IDG and other healthcare providers
- Care plan oversight
- Skilled assessment and support of the patient, family, and caregiver's coping skills
- Medication management
- Home medical equipment as indicated
- Interventions of symptoms directed toward comfort and palliation
- Comfort measures of backrub and hand or other therapeutic massage
- Presence and support
- Volunteer support to patient and family per their request
- Other interventions, based on patient/family needs

## *Safety and Mobility Considerations*

- Providing caregiver with home safety information and instruction related to _____
- Teaching family regarding safety of patient in home
- Teaching family regarding energy conservation techniques
- Teaching safe oral intake (especially liquids)
- Monitoring for choking/aspiration if oral intake is possible
- Teaching caregiver safe and effective suctioning of patient secretions
- Teaching caregiver/family safety related to bed mobility and transfers
- Other interventions, based on patient/family needs

## Emotional/Spiritual Considerations

- Psychosocial assessment of patient and family regarding disease and prognosis (may be completed by the RN or the hospice social worker)
- Emotional support to patient and family with _____, and illness of a terminal nature
- Assessment of mental status and sleep disturbance changes
- Assessment for signs/symptoms of depression
- Spiritual counseling/support offered to patients and caregiver who verbalize emotional or spiritual pain and turmoil
- Support to patient and family/caregivers
- Other interventions, based on patient/family needs

## Skin Considerations

**Assess**

- Assessment and observation of skin integrity and patient's physical status
- Observation and assessment/evaluation of any wound and surrounding skin
- Evaluation of patient's need for equipment/supplies to decrease pressure; alternating pressure mattress, gel foam seat cushion, and heel and elbow protectors
- Observing and applying skilled assessment of areas for possible breakdown, including bony prominences and other pressure-prone areas

**Teach Patient and Family/Caregiver**

- Skin care related to patient's needs, including that of frequent position changes, appropriate pressure pads and mattresses, effective use of turn/pull sheet to avoid friction, skin tears and burns, and the prevention of breakdown
- Proper body alignment and positioning in bed to prevent skin tears from shearing skin

**Provide Care**

- Palliative wound care that focuses on relieving suffering and improving the patient's quality of life when their wound no longer responds to, or the patient can no longer tolerate, curative treatment; palliative wound care concentrates on symptom management, addressing the problems of infection, pain, wound odor, exudate, and decreased self-confidence in end-of-life care (Wound Source, 2017)

## Elimination Considerations

- Assessing bowel regimen, and implement program as needed
- Monitoring bowel patterns, including frequency of bowel movements, and evaluating bowel regimen (for example, stool softeners, laxatives, and dietary changes)
- Checking for and removing impaction per physician orders
- Teaching caregiver daily catheter care and equipment care and signs and symptoms that necessitate calling the hospice
- Changing catheter (specifying type, size, and frequency) as indicated
- Assessing amount and frequency of urinary output
- Other interventions, based on patient/family needs

## Hydration/Nutrition

- Assessing and monitoring hydration/nutrition status
- Providing diet counseling for patient with cachexia
- Teaching family/caregivers proper care of the feeding tube
- Supporting nutrition/hydration by offering patient's choice of favorite or desired foods or liquids
- Maintaining nutrition/hydration by offering patient high-protein diet and food of choice as tolerated
- Teaching patient and family to expect decreased nutritional and fluid intake as disease progresses

- Monitoring and recording weights as ordered
- Other interventions, based on patient/family needs

### Therapeutic/Medication Regimens

- Completing an assessment and reconciliation of all patient prescriptions and over-the-counter drugs, herbal remedies, and other alternative treatments that could affect drug therapy, including, but not limited to, identification of the following:
  - Effectiveness of drug therapy
  - Drug side effects
  - Actual or potential drug interactions
  - Duplicate drug therapy
  - Drug therapy currently associated with laboratory monitoring
- Instruction on all medications, including schedule, functions of specific drugs, and their side effects/interactions
- Monitoring and assessing complications for new medication regimen
- Managing medications-related drug/drug, drug/food side effects
- Monitoring patient's response to medications for pain and symptom control
- Monitoring adherence to medication regimen
- Assessing the patient's unique response to treatments or interventions, and reporting changes or unfavorable responses or reactions to the physician
- Teaching new pain and symptom control medication regimen
- Teaching patient and family about new medications and side effects
- Obtaining venipuncture as ordered every _____ (order frequency)
- Teaching patient and caregiver use of PCA pump
- Assessment for electrolyte imbalance

- Providing nonpharmacological interventions such as progressive muscle relaxation, imagery, positive visualization, music, massage and touch, and humor therapy of patient's choice
- Other interventions, based on patient/family needs

## Other Considerations

- Assessment of disease progression
- Assisting family in setting up patient-centered routine and stressing the importance of adhering to the routine once it is established
- Assessment of the patient's response to treatments and interventions and reporting to the physician any changes, unfavorable responses, or reactions
- Other interventions, based on patient/family needs

## Hospice Aide

- Effective and safe personal care
- Safe ADL assistance and support, ambulation, and transfers
- Observing and reporting any changes in patient condition
- Preparation or assistance with preparation of meals
- Homemaker services (as requested by family)
- Comfort care measures per patient needs and aide care plan
- Other duties as assigned and within the scope of practice

## Social Worker

- Completion of psychosocial assessment
- Support to patient and family/caregivers related to adjusting to the illness and its implications and the need for care
- Identification of optimal coping strategies
- Performing financial assessment and counseling regarding food acquisition and ability to prepare meals

- Interventions/support related to terminal illness and loss
- Emotional/spiritual support
- Facilitation of communication among patient, family, and hospice team
- Referrals/linkage to community services and resources as indicated
- Grief counseling and intervention/support related to illness/loss
- Identification of any illness-related psychiatric condition necessitating care
- Assistance with funeral and burial planning

**Volunteer(s)**

- Support, friendship, companionship, and presence
- Comfort and dignity for patient and family
- Assistance with errands and transportation
- Other services based on interdisciplinary group recommendations and patient/caregiver needs

**Spiritual Counselor**

- Spiritual assessment and care
- Counseling, interventions, and support related to life's meaning (consistent with patient's beliefs)
- Prayer with or for the patient's family using prayers familiar to patient's religious background (per their wishes)
- Support, listening, and presence
- Participation in sacred or spiritual rituals or practices
- Assistance with funeral planning
- Other supportive care, based on patient/family needs and belief systems

## 6. PATIENT, FAMILY, AND CAREGIVER EDUCATIONAL NEEDS

Educational needs are the care regimens that contribute to safe and effective care at home between the hospice team's visits. These include the following:

- The basic tenets of hospice and the availability of support 24 hours a day, 7 days a week
- Home safety assessment and counseling
- Safe and proper body mechanics to promote patient comfort and prevent caregiver safety problems
- Support groups available to the patient's family, such as caregiver support groups
- Skin care regimens
- Catheter and wound care programs
- Effective personal hygiene habits
- Home exercise program, including range of motion
- Safety measures in the home when the patient is immobilized
- Infection control and prevention
- Medication regimen and the medications' relationships to each other
- Importance of medical follow-up
- When to call the hospice
- Anticipated disease progression
- Other information based on the patient's/family's unique needs

## 7. TIPS FOR SUPPORTING QUALITY, SAFETY, AND ELIGIBILITY

- Know that the Medicare Hospice Benefit does not require that the patient be homebound or have identified skilled needs, but care must be medically necessary to qualify for Medicare reimbursement.

- Understand that, unless the patient has a hospice benefit, some insurers will not pay for a skilled nurse visit that is made at death if the patient is dead when the nurse arrives at the home.
- Should the patient's status deteriorate and increased personal care be needed, obtain a verbal order for the increased service, noting frequency and estimating the duration.
- Obtain a verbal order for all medication and skilled treatment changes (for example, antibiotic therapy), and document these in the clinical record.
- Document the symptoms and clinical assessment findings that support the terminal prognosis.
  - Patient changes, symptoms, and clinical information identified from visits and team meetings that support hospice care and limited life expectancy
    - Mentation, behavioral, and cognitive changes
    - Dysphagia, weight loss, dyspnea, infection, sepsis, and new or changed medications
    - Skin changes (for example, inflamed, painful, weeping skin site[s]) and reddened bony prominences
    - Dehydration
    - Patient change and decline
    - Pain, other symptoms not controlled
    - Status after acute episode of _____ (specify)
    - Positive urine, sputum culture; patient started
    - Febrile at _____, pulse change at _____, irregularly irregular
    - Medication adjustments
    - Nutrition, hydration, or elimination concerns (for example, decreased intake, fecal impaction)
    - Any variances to expected outcomes
    - Inability to perform ADLs, personal care
    - Frequent communication required with physician regarding _____ (specify)

- Clearly support the rationale that explains the progression of the illness from the chronic to the terminal stages.

- Coordinate services and consultations with other members of the IDG.

- Document all IDG meetings and communications in the POC and in the progress notes of the clinical record.

- Document coordination of services or consultation providers, such as skilled nursing facility or nursing home staff, inpatient team members, and hired caregivers.

- Document what the patient looks like (frail, pale, poor intake, shortness of breath, inability to do ADLs, and so on).

- Ensure that all team members have provided input into the patient's POC and documented their interventions and goals.

- Remember that the clinical documentation is vital to measuring compliance for quality and reimbursement purposes. Care coordination, timely verbal and initial physician orders, and assessment and addressing of spiritual and psychosocial needs should be clearly documented in the patient's clinical record.

- Make sure that the documentation maintains that all hospice care supports comfort and dignity while meeting patient/family needs.

- Ensure that all team members, including clinicians and social workers, assess, identify, and "hear" spiritual needs that the patient/family want to be addressed. These spiritual issues are important to the provision of quality hospice care and cannot be addressed effectively and promptly by the spiritual counselor alone.

- Remember that the "litmus test" of care coordination rests on the quality of the clinical documentation completed by all team members. Review one of your patient's clinical records and ask yourself the following:

  "If I was unable to give a verbal report/update on this patient, would a peer be able to pick up and provide the same level of care and know (from the documentation) the current orders, including specific medications and other details that contribute to effective hospice care?"

## 8. QUALITY METRICS

- Are the patient's pain and other symptoms managed adequately?
- Is the patient's anxiety managed adequately?
- Is the patient's functional ability/status clearly documented?
- What is the condition of the patient's skin?
- Has the interdisciplinary POC been updated as changes occur and by all interdisciplinary group members?
- Are interventions providing comfort and maintaining dignity?

# NEUROLOGIC DISEASE CARE

## 1. GENERAL CONSIDERATIONS

Neurological conditions are associated with impairments, activity limitations, and disability. Their impact on any given individual depends on the individual's overall health status. Neurological disease may progress in many ways, specific to the disease and the individual. This presents a challenge for care throughout the disease progression and particularly at the end of life. These challenges include the unpredictability of disease progression, associated cognitive change, complex treatments, and concerns and problems encountered with genetically linked diseases. Neurological diseases that are commonly seen in hospice are amyotrophic lateral sclerosis (ALS) and Parkinson's disease, multiple sclerosis (MS), and Huntington's disease. Refer also to the Care Guideline for Alzheimer's disease and other dementias care, earlier in this part. This does not mean that other neurologically based diseases cannot benefit from hospice care; the patient just needs to have an illness that is in its terminal stage and a prognosis of 6 months or less (Palmetto GBA, 2017).

## 2. ELIGIBILITY CONSIDERATIONS

Neurological conditions may support a prognosis of 6 months or less under many clinical scenarios. Medicare regulations require documentation of sufficient "clinical information and other documentation" to support the certification of individuals as having a terminal illness with a life expectancy of 6 or fewer months, if the illness runs its normal course. The identification of specific structural/functional impairments, together with any relevant activity limitations, should serve as the basis for palliative interventions and care planning. General indications for hospice eligibility could include:

- Significant dysphagia
- Aspiration pneumonia
- Recurrent infections—particularly serious respiratory or urinary infections (for example, phelonephritis)

- Marked decline in physical status—generalized weakness and reduced mobility and activity
- Cognitive difficulties—confusion or understated cognitive change
- Weight loss
- Significant compound symptoms:
  - Pain
  - Spasticity
  - Nausea

When addressing neurological diseases, refer to your MAC or other regulatory bodies for up-to-date and specific guidance.

## 3. POTENTIAL DIAGNOSES ICD-10-CM DIAGNOSTIC CODING

The *International Statistical Classification of Diseases and Related Health Problems* 10th Revision (ICD-10-CM) is a coding of diseases and signs, symptoms, abnormal findings, complaints, social circumstances, and external causes of injury or diseases, as classified by the WHO. The following diagnoses and codes are some of the most common conditions seen in this diagnosis. There are specific coding rules and conventions in the official coding manual that must be followed, and these rules may not be included in online websites or EMR software. Consult with a credentialed coder for any questions related to accurate coding.

Neurological disease codes are in the ICD-10-CM manual in Chapter VI—"Diseases of the Nervous System" (G00–G99).

G12.21—Amyotrophic lateral sclerosis

G20—Parkinson's disease

G35—Multiple sclerosis

G10—Huntington's disease

G32.89—Other specified degenerative disorders of nervous system in diseases classified elsewhere

# 4. SAFETY CONSIDERATIONS

- Infection control and prevention/standard precautions (that is, disposal of soiled dressings)
- Side rail use and positioning
- Comprehensive skin care and assessment
- Proper positioning and frequent position changes (for physical safety and skin care)
- Nightlight
- Removal of scatter rugs
- Tub rail, grab bars for bathroom safety
- Smoking and oxygen safety
- Wheelchair/fall precautions
- Home medical equipment safety, including oxygen
- Supportive nonskid shoes and caution on slippery walking surfaces
- Smoke detector and fire evacuation plan
- Supervised care and medication regimen
- Assistance with transfers and ambulation
- Others, based on the patient's unique condition and environment

# 5. SKILLS AND SERVICES IDENTIFIED

## Registered Nurse

**Assess**

Comprehensive assessment of the neurological system including:

- Interview/assessment to identify presence of:
  - Headache
  - Difficulty with speech
  - Inability to read or write
  - Alteration in memory
  - Altered consciousness

- Confusion or change in thinking
- Disorientation
- Decrease in sensation, tingling, or pain
- Motor weakness or decreased strength
- Decreased sense of smell or taste
- Change in vision or diplopia
- Difficulty with swallowing
- Decreased hearing
- Altered gait or balance
- Dizziness
- Seizures, tremors, twitches, or increased tone
- Assessment of level of consciousness
- Assessment of pupillary reaction
- Complete comprehensive assessment of cardiac, respiratory, integumentary, and genitourinary and gastrointestinal systems to determine changes that may indicate decline

### Comfort and Symptom Management

**Assess**

- Complete initial and comprehensive assessment of all systems of patient admitted to hospice for _____ (specify problem necessitating care)
- Assessment of vital signs every visit
- Assessment of fatigue level and its impact on ADLs
- Assessment for depression
- Assessment of mobility and appropriate use of assistive devices
- Assessment of patient, family, and caregiver wishes and expectations regarding care
- Assessment of patient, family, and caregiver resources available for care

- Assessment of pain and other symptoms, including site, duration, characteristics; evaluation of the pain management's effectiveness; identification of need for change, addition, or other plan or dose adjustment

## Teach Patient and Family/Caregiver

- Presentation of hospice philosophy and services
- Explanation of patient rights and responsibilities
- Teaching physical care of patient
- Teaching about specific disease and management at end of life
- Teaching symptom control and relief measures
- Teaching care of weak, terminally ill patient
- Instruction in pain control measures and medications
- Teaching about realistic expectations of disease process
- Teaching care of the dying and identification of signs/symptoms of impending death

## Provide Care/Case Management

- Comprehensive care coordination with all members of the IDG and other healthcare providers
- Care plan oversight
- Skilled assessment and support of the patient, family, and caregiver's coping skills
- Medication management
- Home medical equipment as indicated
- Interventions of symptoms directed toward comfort and palliation
- Comfort measures of backrub and hand or other therapeutic massage
- Presence and support
- Volunteer support to patient and family per their request
- Other interventions, based on patient/family needs

## *Safety and Mobility Considerations*

- Providing caregiver with home safety information and instruction related to _____
- Teaching family regarding safety of patient in home
- Teaching family regarding bleeding precautions for patients on anticoagulant therapy
- Teaching family regarding energy conservation techniques
- Teaching safe oral intake (especially liquids)
- Monitoring for choking/aspiration
- Teaching caregiver safe and effective suctioning of patient secretions
- Teaching caregiver/family safety related to bed mobility and transfers
- Other interventions, based on patient/family needs

## *Emotional/Spiritual Considerations*

- Psychosocial assessment of patient and family regarding disease and prognosis (may be completed by the RN or the hospice social worker)
- Emotional support to patient and family with _____, and illness of a terminal nature
- Assessment of mental status and sleep disturbance changes
- Assessment for signs/symptoms of depression
- Spiritual counseling/support offered to patients and caregiver who verbalize emotional or spiritual pain and turmoil
- Support to patient and family/caregivers
- Other interventions, based on patient/family needs

## *Skin Considerations*

**Assess**

- Assessment and observation of skin integrity and patient's physical status

- Observation and assessment/evaluation of any wound and surrounding skin
- Evaluation of patient's need for equipment/supplies to decrease pressure; alternating pressure mattress, gel foam seat cushion, and heel and elbow protectors
- Observation and assessment of areas for possible breakdown, including bony prominences and other pressure-prone areas

## Teach Patient and Family/Caregiver

- Skin care related to patient's needs, including the need for frequent position changes, appropriate pressure pads and mattresses, effective use of turn/pull sheet to avoid friction, skin tears and burns, and the prevention of breakdown
- Proper body alignment and positioning in bed to prevent skin tears from shearing skin

## Provide Care

- Palliative wound care that focuses on relieving suffering and improving the patient's quality of life when the wound no longer responds to, or the patient can no longer tolerate, curative treatment; palliative wound care concentrates on symptom management, addressing the problems of infection, pain, wound odor, exudate, and decreased self-confidence in end-of-life care (Wound Source, 2017)
- Other interventions, based on patient/family needs

## *Elimination Considerations*

- Assessing bowel regimen, and implementing program as needed
- Monitoring bowel patterns, including frequency of bowel movements, and evaluating bowel regimen (for example, stool softeners, laxatives, and dietary changes)
- Checking for and removing impaction per physician orders
- Implementing bladder training program

- Teaching caregiver daily catheter care and equipment care and signs and symptoms that necessitate calling the hospice
- Changing catheter (specify type, size, and frequency) as indicated
- Assessing amount and frequency of urinary output
- Other interventions, based on patient/family needs

### Hydration/Nutrition

- Assessing and monitoring hydration/nutrition status
- Providing diet counseling for patient with cachexia
- Teaching family/caregivers proper care of the feeding tube
- Supporting nutrition/hydration by offering patient's choice of favorite or desired foods or liquids
- Maintaining nutrition/hydration by offering patient high-protein diet and food of choice as tolerated
- Teaching patient and family to expect decreased nutritional and fluid intake as disease progresses
- Monitoring and recording weights as ordered
- Other interventions, based on patient/family needs

### Therapeutic/Medication Regimens

- Completing an assessment and reconciliation of all patient prescriptions and over-the-counter drugs, herbal remedies, and other alternative treatments that could affect drug therapy, including, but not limited to, identification of the following:
  - Effectiveness of drug therapy
  - Drug side effects
  - Actual or potential drug interactions
  - Duplicate drug therapy
  - Drug therapy currently associated with laboratory monitoring
- Instructing on all medications including schedule, functions of specific drugs, and their side effects/interactions

- Monitoring and assessing complications for new medication regimen
- Managing medications-related drug/drug, drug/food side effects
- Monitoring patient's response to medications for pain and symptom control
- Monitoring adherence to medication regimen
- Assessing the patient's unique response to treatments or interventions, and reporting changes or unfavorable responses or reactions to the physician
- Teaching new pain and symptom control medication regimen
- Teaching patient and family about new medications and side effects
- Obtaining venipuncture as ordered every _____ (order frequency)
- Teaching patient and caregiver use of PCA pump
- Assessing electrolyte imbalance
- Providing nonpharmacological interventions such as progressive muscle relaxation, imagery, positive visualization, music, massage and touch, and humor therapy of patient's choice
- Other interventions, based on patient/family needs

## Other Considerations

- Assessing disease progression
- Assisting family in setting up patient-centered routine and stressing the importance of adhering to the routine once established
- Assessing the patient's response to treatments and interventions and reporting to the physician any changes, unfavorable responses, or reactions
- Other interventions, based on patient/family needs

## Hospice Aide

- Providing effective and safe personal care
- Ensuring safe ADL assistance and support, ambulation and transfers

- Observing for and reporting any changes in patient condition
- Preparing or assisting with preparation of meals
- Providing homemaker services (as requested by family)
- Providing comfort care measures per patient needs and aide care plan
- Other duties as assigned and within the scope of practice

## Social Worker

- Completion of psychosocial assessment
- Support to patient and family/caregivers related to adjusting to the illness and its implications and the need for care
- Identification of optimal coping strategies
- Financial assessment and counseling regarding food acquisition and ability to prepare meals
- Interventions/support related to terminal illness and loss
- Emotional/spiritual support
- Facilitation of communication among patient, family, and hospice team
- Referrals/linkage to community services and resources as indicated
- Grief counseling and intervention/support related to illness/loss
- Identification of any illness-related psychiatric condition necessitating care
- Assistance with funeral and burial planning

## Volunteer(s)

- Support, friendship, companionship, and presence
- Comfort and dignity for patient and family
- Assistance with errands and transportation
- Other services based on interdisciplinary group recommendations and patient/caregiver needs

**Spiritual Counselor**

- Spiritual assessment and care
- Counseling, interventions, and support related to life's meaning (consistent with patient's beliefs)
- Prayer with or for the patient's family using prayers familiar to patient's religious background (per their wishes)
- Support, listening, and presence
- Participation in sacred or spiritual rituals or practices
- Assistance with funeral planning
- Other supportive care, based on patient/family needs and belief systems

## Other Services

- Physical therapy, occupational therapy, and speech therapy as directed by a physician
- Nonpharmacological interventions such as progressive muscle relaxation, imagery, positive visualization, music, massage and touch, pet therapy (including patient's pets if available), and humor therapy of patient's choice
- Plans to engage patient and support comfort, quality, enjoyment, and dignity
- Evaluation and interventions based on patient's and caregiver's unique wishes and needs that support care, comfort, and death in the setting of the patient's choice when possible

## 6. PATIENT, FAMILY, AND CAREGIVER EDUCATIONAL NEEDS

Educational needs are the care regimens that contribute to safe and effective care at home between the hospice team's visits. These include the following:

- The basic tenets of hospice and the availability of support 24 hours a day, 7 days a week

- Home safety assessment and counseling
- Safe and proper body mechanics to promote patient comfort and prevent caregiver safety problems
- Support groups available to the patient's family, such as caregiver support groups
- Skin care regimens
- Catheter and wound care programs
- Effective personal hygiene habits
- Home exercise program, including range of motion
- Safety measures in the home when the patient is immobilized
- Infection control and prevention
- Medication regimen and the medications' relationships to each other
- Importance of medical follow-up
- When to call the hospice
- Anticipated disease progression
- Other information based on the patient's/family's unique needs

## 7. TIPS FOR QUALITY, SAFETY, ELIGIBILITY, AND REIMBURSEMENT

- Know that the Medicare Hospice Benefit does not require that the patient be homebound or have identified skilled needs, but care must be medically necessary to qualify for Medicare reimbursement.
- Understand that, unless the patient has a hospice benefit, some insurers will not pay for a skilled nurse visit that is made at death if the patient is dead when the nurse arrives at the home.
- Should the patient's status deteriorate and increased personal care be needed, obtain a verbal order for the increased service, noting frequency and estimating the duration.

- Obtain a verbal order for all medication and skilled treatment changes (for example, antibiotic therapy), and document these in the clinical record.

- Document the symptoms and clinical assessment findings that support the terminal prognosis:

  - Patient changes, symptoms, and clinical information identified from visits and team meetings that support hospice care and limited life expectancy

    - Mentation, behavioral, and cognitive changes

    - Dysphagia, weight loss, dyspnea, infection, sepsis, and new or changed medications

    - Skin changes (for example, inflamed, painful, weeping skin site[s]) and reddened bony prominences

    - Dehydration

    - Patient change and decline

    - Pain, other symptoms not controlled

    - Status after acute episode of _____ (specify)

    - Positive urine, sputum culture; patient started

    - Febrile at _____, pulse change at _____, irregularly irregular

    - Medication adjustments

    - Nutrition, hydration, or elimination concerns (for example, decreased intake, fecal impaction)

    - Any variances to expected outcomes

    - Inability to perform ADLs, personal care

    - Frequent communication required with physician regarding _____ (specify)

  - Clearly support the rationale that explains the progression of the illness from the chronic to the terminal stages.

  - Coordinate services and consultations with other members of the IDG.

- Document all IDG meetings and communications in the POC and in the progress notes of the clinical record.

- Document coordination of services or consultation providers, such as skilled nursing facility or nursing home staff, inpatient team members, and hired caregivers.

- Document what the patient looks like (frail, pale, poor intake, shortness of breath, inability to do ADLs, and so on).

- Ensure that all team members have provided input into the patient's POC and documented their interventions and goals.

- Remember that the clinical documentation is vital to measuring compliance for quality and reimbursement purposes. Care coordination, timely verbal and initial physician orders, and assessment and addressing of spiritual and psychosocial needs should be clearly documented in the patient's clinical record.

- Make sure that the documentation maintains that all hospice care supports comfort and dignity while meeting patient/family needs.

- Ensure that all team members, including clinicians and social workers, assess, identify, and "hear" spiritual needs that the patient/family want to be addressed. These spiritual issues are important to the provision of quality hospice care and cannot be addressed effectively and promptly by the spiritual counselor alone.

- Remember that the "litmus test" of care coordination rests on the quality of the clinical documentation completed by all team members. Review one of your patient's clinical records and ask yourself the following:

  "If I was unable to give a verbal report/update on this patient, would a peer be able to pick up and provide the same level of care and know (from the documentation) the current orders, including specific medications and other details that contribute to effective hospice care?"

## 8. QUALITY METRICS

- Are the patient's pain and other symptoms managed adequately?
- Is the patient's functional ability/status clearly documented?
- What is the condition of the patient's skin?
- Has the interdisciplinary POC been updated as changes occur and by all interdisciplinary group members?
- Are interventions providing comfort and maintaining dignity?

# PULMONARY CARE

## 1. GENERAL CONSIDERATIONS

Patients and their family members may be referred to hospice care after long battles with chronic pulmonary diseases such as chronic obstructive pulmonary disease (COPD), asthma, bronchitis, and tuberculosis. Care is directed toward controlling and reducing the symptoms of the specific lung pathology. Supportive and skillful care is directed toward comfort and relief of coughing, dyspnea, feelings of tightness, and other complaints and problems.

## 2. ELIGIBILITY CONSIDERATIONS

Patients are considered to be in the terminal stage of pulmonary disease (various forms of advanced pulmonary disease) if they meet the following criteria.

- Severe chronic lung disease characterized as disabling dyspnea at rest, poor or unresponsive to bronchodilators, resulting in decreased functional capacity; for example, bed to chair existence, fatigue, and cough
- Progression of end-stage pulmonary disease, as evidenced by increasing visits to the emergency department or hospitalizations for pulmonary infections or respiratory failure or increasing physician home visits prior to initial certification
- Hypoxemia at rest on room air, as evidenced by $pO2 \leq 55$ mmHg; or oxygen saturation $\leq 88\%$, determined either by arterial blood gases or oxygen saturation monitors
- Right heart failure (RHF) secondary to pulmonary disease
- Unintentional progressive weight loss of greater than 10% of body weight over the preceding 6 months
- Resting tachycardia > 100/min (CGS, 2015).

When addressing pulmonary disease, refer to your MAC or other regulatory bodies for up-to-date and specific guidance.

## 3. POTENTIAL DIAGNOSES ICD-10-CM DIAGNOSTIC CODING

The *International Statistical Classification of Diseases and Related Health Problems* 10th Revision (ICD-10-CM) is a coding of diseases and signs, symptoms, abnormal findings, complaints, social circumstances, and external causes of injury or diseases, as classified by the WHO. There are specific coding rules and conventions in the official coding manual that must be followed, and these rules may not be included in online websites or EMR software. Consult with a credentialed coder for any questions related to accurate coding.

ICD-10-CM Chapter X: "Diseases of the Respiratory System" (J00–J99) contains pulmonary codes.

> J40–J47 Chronic lower respiratory diseases
>
> J20–J22 Other acute lower respiratory infections
>
> J80–J84 Other respiratory diseases principally affecting the interstitium

## 4. SAFETY CONSIDERATIONS

- Infection control and prevention/standard precautions
- Supervised medication administration
- Multiple medications safety (side effects, interactions, storage)
- Home medical equipment safety
- Nightlight
- Removal of scatter rugs
- Tub rail, grab bars for bathroom safety
- Supportive and nonskid shoes
- Smoking and oxygen safety
- Handrail on stairs
- Fall precautions
- Protective skin measures

- Use of handrails
- Smoke detector and fire evacuation plan
- Assistance with ambulation
- Supervised care and medication regimen
- Others, based on the patient's unique condition and environment

## 5. SKILLS AND SERVICES IDENTIFIED

## Registered Nurse

### Assess

- Initial and comprehensive assessment of all systems of patient admitted to hospice for _____ (specify problem necessitating care)
- Comprehensive assessment of the pulmonary system including:
  - Visual inspection—Many abnormalities can be detected by merely observing the chest as the patient is breathing.
  - Auscultation—Listen for the quality and intensity of breath sounds to determine the rate, the rhythm, and whether breath is full and easily audible or diminished. Listen for abnormal breath sounds; these are distinguished from the variations of normal breath sounds that can occur due to hypoventilation or hyperventilation.
    - Abnormal breath sounds are classified into the following categories:
      - Rales: discontinuous sound (crackle)
      - Rhonchus: continuous sound (wheezes)
      - Crackles (course and fine)
      - Wheezes (continuous musical sounds)
- Assessing dyspnea, including the effects of dyspnea on activity and quality of life
- Assessing oxygen saturation and skin color
- Assessing Cor Pulmonale (increased jugular-venous pressure, ascites, jaundice, abnormal heart sounds)

- Assessing signs/symptoms of respiratory infections, including changes in mental status
- Assessing fatigue level and its impact on ADLs and mood
- Assessing mobility and appropriate use of assistive devices
- Assessing vital signs every visit
- Assessing heart rate and rhythm and strength of heartbeat
- Assessing edema, including site and degree
- Assessing patient, family, and caregiver wishes and expectations regarding care
- Assessing patient, family, and caregiver resources available for care
- Assessing pain and other symptoms, including site, duration, and characteristics; evaluating the pain management's effectiveness; identifying need for change, addition, or another plan or dose adjustment
- Assessing need for home medical equipment, such as bedside commodes
- Assessing and observing skin integrity and patient's physical status
  - Observing and evaluating any wound and surrounding skin
  - Evaluating patient's need for equipment/supplies to decrease pressure; alternating pressure mattress, gel foam seat cushion, and heel and elbow protectors
  - Observing and applying skilled assessment of areas for possible breakdown, including bony prominences, and other pressure-prone areas

### Teach Patient and Family/Caregiver

- Presentation of hospice philosophy and services
- Explanation of patient rights and responsibilities
- Teaching physical care of patient
- Teaching about specific disease and management at end of life
- Teaching symptom control and relief measures for severe shortness of breath, including nonpharmacologic interventions

- Teaching care of weak, terminally ill patient
- Instruction in pain control measures and medications
- Teaching about realistic expectations of disease process
- Teaching care of the dying and identification of signs/symptoms of impending death

**Provide Care/Case Management**

- Comprehensive care coordination with all members of the IDG and other healthcare providers
- Care plan oversight
- Skilled assessment and support of the patient, family, and caregiver's coping skills
- Medication management
- Home medical equipment as indicated
- Interventions of symptoms directed toward comfort and palliation
- Comfort measures of backrub and hand or other therapeutic massage
- Presence and support
- Volunteer support to patient and family per their request
- Other interventions, based on patient/family needs

*Safety and Mobility Considerations*

- Providing caregiver with home safety information and instruction related to _____
- Teaching family regarding safety of patient in home
- Teaching family regarding oxygen safety
- Teaching family regarding energy conservation techniques
- Teaching caregiver/family safety related to bed mobility and transfers
- Other interventions, based on patient/family needs

## Emotional/Spiritual Considerations

- Psychosocial assessment of patient and family regarding disease and prognosis (may be completed by the RN or the hospice social worker)
- Emotional support to patient and family with _____, and illness of a terminal nature
- Assessing mental status and sleep disturbance changes
- Assessing signs/symptoms of depression
- Spiritual counseling/support offered to patients and caregiver who verbalize emotional or spiritual pain and turmoil
- Support to patient and family/caregivers
- Other interventions, based on patient/family needs

## Skin Considerations

**Assess**

- Assessment and observation of skin integrity and patient's physical status
- Observation and assessment/evaluation of any wound and surrounding skin
- Evaluation of patient's need for equipment/supplies to decrease pressure; alternating pressure mattress, gel foam seat cushion, and heel and elbow protectors
- Observation and assessment of areas for possible breakdown, including bony prominences and other pressure-prone areas

**Teach Patient and Family/Caregiver**

- Skin care related to patient's needs, including the need for frequent position changes, appropriate pressure pads and mattresses, effective use of turn/pull sheet to avoid friction, skin tears and burns, and the prevention of breakdown
- Proper body alignment and positioning in bed to prevent skin tears from shearing skin

**Provide Care**

- Palliative wound care that focuses on relieving suffering and improving the patient's quality of life when the wound no longer responds to, or the patient can no longer tolerate, curative treatment; palliative wound care concentrates on symptom management, addressing the problems of infection, pain, wound odor, exudate, and decreased self-confidence in end-of-life care (Wound Source, 2017)
- Other interventions, based on patient/family needs

## Elimination Considerations

- Assessing bowel regimen, and implementing program as needed
- Monitoring bowel patterns, including frequency of bowel movements, and evaluating bowel regimen (for example, stool softeners, laxatives, and dietary changes)
- Checking for and removing impaction per physician orders
- Implementing bladder training program
- Teaching caregiver daily catheter care and equipment care and signs and symptoms that necessitate calling the hospice
- Changing catheter (specify type, size, and frequency) as indicated
- Assessing amount and frequency of urinary output
- Other interventions, based on patient/family needs

## Hydration/Nutrition

- Assessing and monitoring hydration/nutrition status
- Providing diet counseling for patient with cachexia
- Teaching family/caregivers proper care of the feeding tube
- Supporting nutrition/hydration by offering patient's choice of favorite or desired foods or liquids
- Maintaining nutrition/hydration by offering patient high-protein diet and food of choice as tolerated

- Teaching patient and family to expect decreased nutritional and fluid intake as disease progresses
- Monitoring and recording weights as ordered
- Other interventions, based on patient/family needs

## Therapeutic/Medication Regimens

- Completion of an assessment and reconciliation of all patient prescriptions and over-the-counter drugs, herbal remedies, and other alternative treatments that could affect drug therapy, including, but not limited to, identification of the following:
  - Effectiveness of drug therapy
  - Drug side effects
  - Actual or potential drug interactions
  - Duplicate drug therapy
  - Drug therapy currently associated with laboratory monitoring
- Instruction on all medications, including schedule, functions of specific drugs, and their side effects/interactions
- Monitoring and assessing complications for new medication regimen
- Managing medications-related drug/drug, drug/food side effects
- Monitoring patient's response to medications for pain and symptom control
- Monitoring adherence to medication regimen
- Assessing the patient's unique response to treatments or interventions, and reporting changes or unfavorable responses or reactions to the physician
- Teaching new pain and symptom control medication regimen
- Teaching patient and family about new medications and side effects
- Obtaining venipuncture as ordered every _____ (order frequency)
- Teaching patient and caregiver use of PCA pump
- Assessing electrolyte imbalance

- Providing nonpharmacological interventions such as progressive muscle relaxation, imagery, positive visualization, music, massage and touch, and humor therapy of patient's choice
- Other interventions, based on patient/family needs

### Other Considerations

- Assessing disease progression
- Assisting family in setting up patient-centered routine and stressing the importance of adhering to the routine once established
- Assessing the patient's response to treatments and interventions and reporting to the physician any changes, unfavorable responses, or reactions
- Other interventions, based on patient/family needs

### Hospice Aide

- Providing effective and safe personal care
- Ensuring safe ADL assistance and support, ambulation, and transfers
- Observing and reporting any changes in patient condition
- Preparing or assisting with preparation of meals
- Providing homemaker services (as requested by family)
- Providing comfort care measures per patient needs and aide care plan
- Other duties as assigned and within the scope of practice

### Social Worker

- Completion of psychosocial assessment
- Support to patient and family/caregivers related to adjusting to the illness and its implications and the need for care
- Identification of optimal coping strategies
- Financial assessment and counseling regarding food acquisition and ability to prepare meals

- Interventions/support related to terminal illness and loss
- Emotional/spiritual support
- Facilitation of communication among patient, family, and hospice team
- Referrals/linkage to community services and resources as indicated
- Grief counseling and intervention/support related to illness/loss
- Identification of any illness-related psychiatric condition necessitating care
- Assistance with funeral and burial planning

## Volunteer(s)

- Support, friendship, companionship, and presence
- Comfort and dignity for patient and family
- Assistance with errands and transportation
- Other services based on interdisciplinary group recommendations and patient/caregiver needs

## Spiritual Counselor

- Spiritual assessment and care
- Counseling, interventions, and support related to life's meaning (consistent with patient's beliefs)
- Prayer with or for the patient's family using prayers familiar to patient's religious background (per their wishes)
- Support, listening, and presence
- Participation in sacred or spiritual rituals or practices
- Assistance with funeral planning
- Other supportive care, based on patient/family needs and belief systems

## Other Services

- Physical therapy, occupational therapy, and speech therapy as directed by a physician

- Nonpharmacological interventions such as progressive muscle relaxation, imagery, positive visualization, music, massage and touch, pet therapy (including patient's pets if available), and humor therapy of patient's choice
- Plans to engage patient and support comfort, quality, enjoyment, and dignity
- Evaluation and interventions based on patient's and caregiver's unique wishes and needs that support care, comfort, and death in the setting of the patient's choice when possible

## 6. PATIENT, FAMILY, AND CAREGIVER EDUCATIONAL NEEDS

Educational needs are the care regimens that contribute to safe and effective care at home between the hospice team's visits. These include the following:

- The basic tenets of hospice and the availability of support 24 hours a day, 7 days a week
- Home safety assessment and counseling
- Safe and proper body mechanics to promote patient comfort and prevent caregiver safety problems
- Support groups available to the patient's family, such as caregiver support groups
- Skin care regimens
- Effective personal hygiene habits
- Home exercise program, including range of motion
- Infection control and prevention
- Medication regimen and the medications' relationships to each other
- Importance of medical follow-up
- Knowledge of when to call hospice
- Anticipated disease progression
- Other information based on the patient's/family's unique needs

## 7. TIPS FOR QUALITY, SAFETY, ELIGIBILITY, AND REIMBURSEMENT

- Know that the Medicare Hospice Benefit does not require that the patient be homebound or have identified skilled needs, but care must be medically necessary to qualify for Medicare reimbursement.

- Understand that, unless the patient has a hospice benefit, some insurers will not pay for a skilled nurse visit that is made at death if the patient is dead when the nurse arrives at the home.

- Should the patient's status deteriorate and increased personal care be needed, obtain a verbal order for the increased service, noting frequency and estimating the duration.

- Obtain a verbal order for all medication and skilled treatment changes (for example, antibiotic therapy), and document these in the clinical record.

- Document the symptoms and clinical assessment findings that support the terminal prognosis.
  - Patient changes, symptoms, and clinical information identified from visits and team meetings that support hospice care and limited life expectancy
    - Mentation, behavioral, and cognitive changes
    - Dysphagia, weight loss, dyspnea, infection, sepsis, and new or changed medications
    - Skin changes (for example, inflamed, painful, weeping skin site[s]) and reddened bony prominences
    - Dehydration
    - Patient change and decline
    - Pain, other symptoms not controlled
    - Status after acute episode of _____ (specify)
    - Positive urine, sputum culture; patient started
    - Febrile at _____, pulse change at _____, irregularly irregular
    - Medication adjustments

- Nutrition, hydration, or elimination concerns (for example, decreased intake, fecal impaction)
- Any variances to expected outcomes
- Inability to perform ADLs, personal care
- Frequent communication required with physician regarding _____ (specify)
  - Clearly support the rationale that explains the progression of the illness from the chronic to the terminal stages.
  - Coordinate services and consultations with other members of the IDG.
- Document all interdisciplinary group meetings and communications in the POC and in the progress notes of the clinical record.
- Document coordination of services or consultation providers, such as skilled nursing facility or nursing home staff, inpatient team members, and hired caregivers.
- Document what the patient looks like (frail, pale, poor intake, shortness of breath, inability to do ADLs, and so on).
- Ensure that all team members have provided input into the patient's POC and documented their interventions and goals.
- Remember that the clinical documentation is vital to measuring compliance for quality and reimbursement purposes. Care coordination, timely verbal and initial physician orders, and assessment and addressing of spiritual and psychosocial needs should be clearly documented in the patient's clinical record.
- Make sure the documentation maintains that all hospice care supports comfort and dignity while meeting patient/family needs.
- Ensure that all team members, including clinicians and social workers, assess, identify, and "hear" spiritual needs that the patient/family want to be addressed. These spiritual issues are important to the provision of quality hospice care and cannot be addressed effectively and promptly by the spiritual counselor alone.

- Remember that the "litmus test" of care coordination rests on the quality of the clinical documentation completed by all team members. Review one of your patient's clinical records and ask yourself the following:

  "If I was unable to give a verbal report/update on this patient, would a peer be able to pick up and provide the same level of care and know (from the documentation) the current orders, including specific medications and other details that contribute to effective hospice care?"

## 8. QUALITY METRICS

- Are the patient's pain, dyspnea, and other symptoms managed adequately?

- Is the patient's functional ability/status clearly documented?

- What is the condition of the patient's skin?

- Has the interdisciplinary POC been updated as changes occur and by all interdisciplinary group members?

- Are interventions providing comfort and maintaining dignity?

# RENAL DISEASE CARE

## 1. GENERAL CONSIDERATIONS

End-stage renal disease (ESRD) occurs when chronic kidney disease reaches an advanced state. With ESRD, a patient needs dialysis or a kidney transplant to stay alive. Patients who opt for a palliative care approach forgo dialysis or transplant and choose conservative care to manage symptoms and achieve the best quality of life possible during their remaining time.

## 2. ELIGIBILITY CONSIDERATIONS

The identification of specific structural/functional impairments, with any relevant activity limitations, should serve as the basis for palliative interventions. The structural and functional impairments associated with a primary diagnosis of ESRD are often complicated by comorbid or secondary conditions (Palmetto GBA, 2017). A patient is eligible for hospice as follows:

- The patient is not seeking dialysis or renal transplant or is discontinuing dialysis.
- Creatinine clearance is < 10 cc/min (< 15 cc/min for diabetics) based on measurement or calculation; or < 15 cc/min (< 20cc/min for diabetics) with comorbidity of congestive heart failure.
- Serum creatinine is > 8.0 mg/dl (> 6.0 mg/dl for diabetics).
- Signs and symptoms of renal failure:
  - Uremia
  - Oliguria (< 400 cc/24 hours)
  - Intractable hyperkalemia (> 7.0) not responsive to treatment
  - Uremic pericarditis
  - Hepatorenal syndrome
  - Intractable fluid overload, not responsive to treatment (CGS, 2015)

When addressing renal disease, refer to your MAC or other regulatory bodies for up-to-date and specific guidance.

## 3. POTENTIAL DIAGNOSES ICD-10-CM DIAGNOSTIC CODING

The *International Statistical Classification of Diseases and Related Health Problems* 10th Revision (ICD-10-CM) is a coding of diseases and signs, symptoms, abnormal findings, complaints, social circumstances, and external causes of injury or diseases, as classified by the WHO. Dementia codes are listed in *Chapter V: Mental and Behavioral Disorders* in the ICD-10-CM coding manual. Refer to the earlier Care Guidelines for Alzheimer's Disease and other dementias care. There are specific coding rules and conventions in the official coding manual that must be followed, and these rules may not be included in online websites or EMR software. Consult with a credentialed coder for any questions related to accurate coding.

RD codes are in the ICD-10-CM in Chapter XIV, "Diseases of the Genitourinary System" (N00–N99).

> N18.6 End-stage renal disease (code must be followed by one or more code(s) that represent the manifestation)
>
> Z99.2 Code to identify dialysis status

## 4. SAFETY CONSIDERATIONS
- Infection control and prevention/standard precautions
- Supervised medication administration
- Multiple medications safety (side effects, interactions, storage)
- Home medical equipment safety, including oxygen
- Nightlight
- Removal of scatter rugs
- Tub rail, grab bars for bathroom safety
- Supportive and nonskid shoes

- Smoking and oxygen safety
- Handrails on stairs
- Fall precautions
- Protective skin measures
- Stairway precautions
- Smoke detector and fire evacuation plan
- Assistance with ambulation
- Supervised care and medication regimen
- Others, based on the patient's unique condition and environment

## 5. SKILLS AND SERVICES IDENTIFIED

## Registered Nurse

### Assess

- Comprehensive assessment of the genitourinary system, gastrointestinal system, integumentary system, and cardiopulmonary systems; signs and symptoms of ESRD include:
  - Nausea
  - Vomiting
  - Loss of appetite
  - Fatigue and weakness
  - Sleep problems
  - Changes in urination
  - Decreased mental sharpness
  - Muscle twitches and cramps
  - Swelling of feet and ankles
  - Persistent itching
  - Chest pain, if fluid builds up around the lining of the heart
  - Shortness of breath, if fluid builds up in the lungs
  - High blood pressure (hypertension) that is difficult to control (Mayo Clinic, 2017b)

- Completion of initial and comprehensive assessment of all systems of patient admitted to hospice for _____ (specify problem necessitating care)
- Assessment of vital signs every visit
- Assessment of patient, family, and caregiver wishes and expectations regarding care
- Assessment of patient, family, and caregiver resources available for care
- Assessment of pain and other symptoms, including site, duration, and characteristics; evaluation of the pain management's effectiveness; identification of the need for change, addition, or another plan or dose adjustment

## Teach Patient and Family/Caregiver

- Presentation of hospice philosophy and services
- Explanation of patient rights and responsibilities
- Teaching physical care of patient
- Teaching about specific disease and management at end of life
- Teaching new pain and symptom control medication regimen
- Teaching symptom control and relief measures
- Teaching care of weak, terminally ill patient
- Instruction in pain control measures and medications
- Teaching about realistic expectations of disease process
- Teaching care of the dying and identification of signs/symptoms of impending death

## Provide Care/Case Management

- Comprehensive care coordination with all members of the IDG and other healthcare providers
- Care plan oversight
- Skilled assessment and support of the patient, family, and caregiver's coping skills

- Medication management
- Home medical equipment as indicated
- Interventions of symptoms directed toward comfort and palliation
- Comfort measures of backrub and hand or other therapeutic massage
- Presence and support
- Volunteer support to patient and family per their request
- Other interventions, based on patient/family needs

## Safety and Mobility Considerations

- Providing caregiver with home safety information and instruction related to _____
- Teaching family regarding safety of patient in home
- Teaching family regarding energy conservation techniques
- Teaching safe oral intake (especially liquids)
- Monitoring for choking/aspiration if oral intake is possible
- Teaching caregiver safe and effective suctioning of patient secretions
- Teaching caregiver/family safety related to bed mobility and transfers
- Performing other interventions, based on patient/family needs

## Emotional/Spiritual Considerations

- Psychosocial assessment of patient and family regarding disease and prognosis (may be completed by the RN or the hospice social worker)
- Emotional support to patient and family with _____, and illness of a terminal nature
- Assessment of mental status and sleep disturbance changes
- Assessment of signs/symptoms of depression

- Spiritual counseling/support offered to patients and caregiver who verbalize emotional or spiritual pain and turmoil
- Support to patient and family/caregivers
- Other interventions, based on patient/family needs

## Skin Considerations

### Assess

- Assessment and observation of skin integrity and patient's physical status
- Observation and assessment/evaluation of any wound and surrounding skin
- Evaluation of patient's need for equipment/supplies to decrease pressure; alternating pressure mattress, gel foam seat cushion, and heel and elbow protectors
- Observation and skilled assessment of areas for possible breakdown, including bony prominences and other pressure-prone areas

### Teach Patient and Family/Caregiver

- Skin care related to patient's needs, including the need for frequent position changes, appropriate pressure pads and mattresses, effective use of turn/pull sheet to avoid friction, skin tears and burns, and the prevention of breakdown
- Proper body alignment and positioning in bed to prevent skin tears from shearing skin

### Provide Care

- Palliative wound care that focuses on relieving suffering and improving the patient's quality of life when the wound no longer responds to, or the patient can no longer tolerate, curative treatment; palliative wound care concentrates on symptom management, addressing the problems of infection, pain, wound odor, exudate, and decreased self-confidence in end-of-life care (Wound Source, 2017)

## Elimination Considerations

- Assessing bowel regimen and implementing program as needed
- Monitoring bowel patterns, including frequency of bowel movements, and evaluating bowel regimen (for example, stool softeners, laxatives, and dietary changes)
- Checking for and removing impaction per physician orders
- Teaching caregiver daily catheter care and equipment care and signs and symptoms that necessitate calling the hospice
- Changing catheter (specifying type, size, and frequency) as indicated
- Assessing amount and frequency of urinary output
- Other interventions, based on patient/family needs

## Hydration/Nutrition

- Assessing and monitoring hydration/nutrition status
- Providing diet counseling for patient with cachexia
- Teaching family/caregivers proper care of the feeding tube
- Supporting nutrition/hydration by offering patient's choice of favorite or desired foods or liquids
- Maintaining nutrition/hydration by offering patient high-protein diet and food of choice as tolerated
- Teaching patient and family to expect decreased nutritional and fluid intake as disease progresses
- Monitoring and recording weights as ordered
- Other interventions, based on patient/family needs

## Therapeutic/Medication Regimens

- Completion of an assessment and reconciliation of all patient prescriptions and over-the-counter drugs, herbal remedies, and other alternative treatments that could affect drug therapy, including, but not limited to, identification of the following:
  - Effectiveness of drug therapy
  - Drug side effects

- • Actual or potential drug interactions
- • Duplicate drug therapy
- • Drug therapy currently associated with laboratory monitoring
- Instruction on all medications including schedule, functions of specific drugs, and their side effects/interactions
- Monitoring and assessing complications for new medication regimen
- Managing medications-related drug/drug, drug/food side effects
- Monitoring patient's response to medications for pain and symptom control
- Monitoring adherence to medication regimen
- Assessing the patient's unique response to treatments or interventions, and reporting changes or unfavorable responses or reactions to the physician
- Teaching new pain and symptom control medication regimen
- Teaching patient and family about new medications and side effects
- Obtaining venipuncture as ordered every _____ (order frequency)
- Teaching patient and caregiver use of PCA pump
- Assessing electrolyte imbalance
- Providing nonpharmacological interventions such as progressive muscle relaxation, imagery, positive visualization, music, massage and touch, and humor therapy of patient's choice
- Other interventions, based on patient/family needs

## Other Considerations

- Assessing disease progression
- Assisting family in setting up patient-centered routine and stressing the importance of adhering to the routine once established
- Assessing the patient's response to treatments and interventions and reporting to the physician any changes, unfavorable responses, or reactions
- Other interventions, based on patient/family needs

**Hospice Aide**

- Effective and safe personal care
- Safe ADL assistance and support, ambulation, and transfers
- Observation and report of any changes in patient condition
- Preparation or assistance with preparation of meals
- Homemaker services (as requested by family)
- Comfort care measures per patient needs and aide care plan
- Other duties as assigned and within the scope of practice

**Social Worker**

- Completion of psychosocial assessment
- Support to patient and family/caregivers related to adjusting to the illness and its implications and the need for care
- Identification of optimal coping strategies
- Financial assessment and counseling regarding food acquisition and ability to prepare meals
- Interventions/support related to terminal illness and loss
- Emotional/spiritual support
- Facilitation of communication among patient, family, and hospice team
- Referrals/linkage to community services and resources as indicated
- Grief counseling and intervention/support related to illness/loss
- Identification of any illness-related psychiatric condition necessitating care
- Assistance with funeral and burial planning

**Volunteer(s)**

- Support, friendship, companionship, and presence
- Comfort and dignity for patient and family
- Assistance with errands and transportation
- Other services based on interdisciplinary group recommendations and patient/caregiver needs

**Spiritual Counselor**

- Spiritual assessment and care
- Counseling, interventions, and support related to life's meaning (consistent with patient's beliefs)
- Prayer with or for the patient's family using prayers familiar to patient's religious background (per their wishes)
- Support, listening, and presence
- Participation in sacred or spiritual rituals or practices
- Assistance with funeral planning
- Other supportive care, based on patient/family needs and belief systems

### Other Services

- Physical therapy, occupational therapy, and speech therapy as directed by a physician
- Nonpharmacological interventions such as progressive muscle relaxation, imagery, positive visualization, music, massage and touch, pet therapy (including patient's pets if available), and humor therapy of patient's choice
- Plans to engage patient and support comfort, quality, enjoyment, and dignity
- Evaluation and interventions based on patient's and caregiver's unique wishes and needs that support care, comfort, and death in the setting of the patient's choice when possible

## 6. PATIENT, FAMILY, AND CAREGIVER EDUCATIONAL NEEDS

Educational needs are the care regimens that contribute to safe and effective care at home between the hospice team's visits. These include the following:

- The basic tenets of hospice and the availability of support 24 hours a day, 7 days a week

- Home safety assessment and counseling
- Safe and proper body mechanics to promote patient comfort and prevent caregiver safety problems
- Support groups available to the patient's family, such as caregiver support groups
- Skin care regimens
- Catheter and wound care programs
- Effective personal hygiene habits
- Home exercise program, including range of motion
- Safety measures in the home when the patient is immobilized
- Infection control and prevention
- Medication regimen and the medications' relationships to each other
- Importance of medical follow-up
- When to call the hospice
- Anticipated disease progression
- Other information based on the patient's/family's unique needs

## 7. TIPS FOR SUPPORTING QUALITY, SAFETY, AND ELIGIBILITY

- Know that the Medicare Hospice Benefit does not require that the patient be homebound or have identified skilled needs, but care must be medically necessary to qualify for Medicare reimbursement.
- Understand that, unless the patient has a hospice benefit, some insurers will not pay for a skilled nurse visit that is made at death if the patient is dead when the nurse arrives at the home.
- Should the patient's status deteriorate and increased personal care be needed, obtain a verbal order for the increased service, noting frequency and estimating the duration.

- Obtain a verbal order for all medication and skilled treatment changes (for example, antibiotic therapy), and document these in the clinical record.
- Document the symptoms and clinical assessment findings that support the terminal prognosis.
  - Patient changes, symptoms, and clinical information identified from visits and team meetings that support hospice care and limited life expectancy
    - Mentation, behavioral, and cognitive changes
    - Dysphagia, weight loss, dyspnea, infection, sepsis, and new or changed medications
    - Skin changes (for example, inflamed, painful, weeping skin site[s]) and reddened bony prominences
    - Dehydration
    - Patient change and decline
    - Pain, other symptoms not controlled
    - Status after acute episode of _____ (specify)
    - Positive urine, sputum culture; patient started
    - Febrile at _____, pulse change at_____, irregularly irregular
    - Medication adjustments
    - Nutrition, hydration, or elimination concerns (for example, decreased intake, fecal impaction)
    - Any variances to expected outcomes
    - Inability to perform ADLs, personal care
    - Frequent communication required with physician regarding _____ (specify)
  - Clearly support the rationale that explains the progression of the illness from the chronic to the terminal stages.
  - Coordinate services and consultations with other members of the IDG.

- Document all interdisciplinary group meetings and communications in the POC and in the progress notes of the clinical record.

- Document coordination of services or consultation providers, such as skilled nursing facility or nursing home staff, inpatient team members, and hired caregivers.

- Document what the patient looks like (frail, pale, poor intake, shortness of breath, inability to do ADLs, and so on).

- Ensure that all team members have provided input into the patient's POC and documented their interventions and goals.

- Remember that the clinical documentation is vital to measuring compliance for quality and reimbursement purposes. Care coordination, timely verbal and initial physician orders, and assessment and addressing of spiritual and psychosocial needs should be clearly documented in the patient's clinical record.

- Make sure that the documentation maintains that all hospice care supports comfort and dignity while meeting patient/family needs.

- Ensure that all team members, including clinicians and social workers, assess, identify, and "hear" spiritual needs that the patient/family want to be addressed. These spiritual issues are important to the provision of quality hospice care and cannot be addressed effectively and promptly by the spiritual counselor alone.

- Remember that the "litmus test" of care coordination rests on the quality of the clinical documentation completed by all team members. Review one of your patient's clinical records and ask yourself the following:

  "If I was unable to give a verbal report/update on this patient, would a peer be able to pick up and provide the same level of care and know (from the documentation) the current orders, including specific medications and other details that contribute to effective hospice care?"

## 8. QUALITY METRICS

- Are the patient's pain and other symptoms managed adequately?
- Is the patient's anxiety managed adequately?
- Is the patient's functional ability/status clearly documented?
- What is the condition of the patient's skin?
- Has the interdisciplinary POC been updated as changes occur and by all interdisciplinary group members?
- Are interventions providing comfort and maintaining dignity?

# References

Anderson, F., Downing, G. M., Hill, J., Casorso, L., & Lerch, N. (1995). Palliative performance scale (PPS): A new tool. *Journal of Palliative Care, 12*(1), 5–11.

Centers for Medicare and Medicaid Services. (2014, August 22). Hospice manual update for diagnosis reporting and filing hospice notice of election (NOE) and termination or revocation of election. Retrieved from https://www.cms.gov/Regulations-and-Guidance/Guidance/Transmittals/downloads/R3032CP.pdf

Centers for Medicare and Medicaid Services. (2015, October). Local coverage determination (LCD): Hospice determining terminal status. Retrieved from https://www.cms.gov/medicare-coverage-database/details/lcd-details.aspx?LCDId=34538&ContrId=236&ver=3&ContrVer=2&CntrctrSelected=236*2&Cntrctr=236&name=+(15004%2c+HHH+MAC)&s=All&DocType=Active%7cFuture&bc=AggAAAQAAAAAAA%3d%3d&

CGS. (2015). Local coverage determination (LCD): Hospice determining terminal status (L34538). Retrieved from https://www.cms.gov/medicare-coverage-database/details/lcd-details.aspx?LCDId=34538&ContrId=236&ver=3&ContrVer=2&CntrctrSelected=236*2&Cntrctr=236&name=+(15004%2c+HHH+MAC)&s=All&DocType=Active%7cFuture&bc=AggAAAQAAAAAAA%3d%3d&

Cox-North, P., Doorenbos, A., Shannon, S. E., Scott, J., & Curtis, J. R. (2013). The transition to end-of-life care in end-stage liver disease. *Journal of Hospice & Palliative Nursing, 15*(4), 209–215.

Mayo Clinic. (2017a). Liver disease. Retrieved from http://www.mayoclinic.org/diseases-conditions/liver-problems/basics/definition/con-20025300

Mayo Clinic. (2017b). End-stage renal disease. Retrieved from http://www.mayoclinic.org/diseases-conditions/end-stage-renal-disease/symptoms-causes/dxc-20211681

National Cancer Institute. (2016, April 8). Last days of life (PDQ)—Health professional version. Retrieved from https://www.cancer.gov/about-cancer/advanced-cancer/caregivers/planning/last-days-hp-pdq#section/_249

Palmetto GBA. (2017, January 1). Local coverage determination (LCD): Hospice Alzheimer's disease & related disorders (L34567). Retrieved from https://www.cms.gov/medicare-coverage-database/details/lcd-details.aspx?LCDId=34567&ContrId=373&ver=16&ContrVer=1&CntrctrSelected=373*1&Cntrctr=373&DocType=Active&s=22&bc=AggAAAQAAAAAAA%3d%3d&

Reisberg, B. (1988). Functional Assessment Staging (FAST). *Psychopharmacology Bulletin, 24*:653–659.

Schag, C. C., Heinrich, R. L., & Ganz, P. A. (1984). Karnofsky performance status revisited: Reliability, validity, and guidelines. *Journal of Clinical Oncology, 2*(3), 187–193.

Wong-Baker Faces Foundation. (2016). Faces of pain care. Retrieved from http://wongbakerfaces.org/

Wound Source. (2017). Palliative wound care. Retrieved from http://www.woundsource.com/patientcondition/palliative-wound-care

# Hospice Conditions of Participation: Subpart B—Eligibility, Election, and Duration of Benefits

**Title 42 Chapter IV Part 418 Subpart B**
**§ 418.20—Eligibility requirements.**

In order to be eligible to elect hospice care under Medicare, an individual must be:

(a) Entitled to Part A of Medicare; and

(b) Certified as being terminally ill in accordance with § 418.22.

**§ 418.21—Duration of hospice care coverage - Election periods.**

(a) Subject to the conditions set forth in this part, an individual may elect to receive hospice care during one or more of the following election periods:

(1) An initial 90-day period;

(2) A subsequent 90-day period; or

(3) An unlimited number of subsequent 60-day periods.

(b)   The periods of care are available in the order listed and may be elected separately at different times.

**[55 FR 50834, Dec. 11, 1990, as amended at 57 FR 36017, Aug. 12, 1992; 70 FR 70546, Nov. 22, 2005]**

**§ 418.22—Certification of terminal illness.**

(a)   *Timing of certification*

(1)   *General rule.* The hospice must obtain written certification of terminal illness for each of the periods listed in § 418.21, even if a single election continues in effect for an unlimited number of periods, as provided in § 418.24(c).

(2)   *Basic requirement.* Except as provided in paragraph (a)(3) of this section, the hospice must obtain the written certification before it submits a claim for payment.

(3)   *Exceptions.*

(i)   If the hospice cannot obtain the written certification within 2 calendar days, after a period begins, it must obtain an oral certification within 2 calendar days and the written certification before it submits a claim for payment.

(ii)   Certifications may be completed no more than 15 calendar days prior to the effective date of election.

(iii)   Recertifications may be completed no more than 15 calendar days prior to the start of the subsequent benefit period.

(4)   *Face-to-face encounter.* As of January 1, 2011, a hospice physician or hospice nurse practitioner must have a face-to-face encounter with each hospice patient whose total stay across all hospices is anticipated to reach the 3rd benefit period. The face-to-face encounter must occur prior to, but no more than 30 calendar days prior to, the 3rd benefit period recertification, and every benefit period recertification thereafter, to gather clinical findings to determine continued eligibility for hospice care.

(b)  *Content of certification.* Certification will be based on the physician's or medical director's clinical judgment regarding the normal course of the individual's illness. The certification must conform to the following requirements:

(1)  The certification must specify that the individual's prognosis is for a life expectancy of 6 months or less if the terminal illness runs its normal course.

(2)  Clinical information and other documentation that support the medical prognosis must accompany the certification and must be filed in the medical record with the written certification as set forth in paragraph (d)(2) of this section. Initially, the clinical information may be provided verbally, and must be documented in the medical record and included as part of the hospice's eligibility assessment.

(3)  The physician must include a brief narrative explanation of the clinical findings that supports a life expectancy of 6 months or less as part of the certification and recertification forms, or as an addendum to the certification and recertification forms.

(i)  If the narrative is part of the certification or recertification form, then the narrative must be located immediately prior to the physician's signature.

(ii)  If the narrative exists as an addendum to the certification or recertification form, in addition to the physician's signature on the certification or recertification form, the physician must also sign immediately following the narrative in the addendum.

(iii)  The narrative shall include a statement directly above the physician signature attesting that by signing, the physician confirms that he/she composed the narrative based on his/her review of the patient's medical record or, if applicable, his/her examination of the patient.

(iv)  The narrative must reflect the patient's individual clinical circumstances and cannot contain check boxes or standard language used for all patients.

      (v) The narrative associated with the 3rd benefit period recertification and every subsequent recertification must include an explanation of why the clinical findings of the face-to-face encounter support a life expectancy of 6 months or less.

   (4) The physician or nurse practitioner who performs the face-to-face encounter with the patient described in paragraph (a)(4) of this section must attest in writing that he or she had a face-to-face encounter with the patient, including the date of that visit. The attestation of the nurse practitioner or a non-certifying hospice physician shall state that the clinical findings of that visit were provided to the certifying physician for use in determining continued eligibility for hospice care.

   (5) All certifications and recertifications must be signed and dated by the physician(s), and must include the benefit period dates to which the certification or recertification applies.

(c) *Sources of certification.*

   (1) For the initial 90-day period, the hospice must obtain written certification statements (and oral certification statements if required under paragraph (a)(3) of this section) from

      (i) The medical director of the hospice or the physician member of the hospice interdisciplinary group; and

      (ii) The individual's attending physician, if the individual has an attending physician. The attending physician must meet the definition of physician specified in § 410.20 of this subchapter.

   (2) For subsequent periods, the only requirement is certification by one of the physicians listed in paragraph (c)(1)(i) of this section.

(d) *Maintenance of records.* Hospice staff must

   (1) Make an appropriate entry in the patient's medical record as soon as they receive an oral certification; and

   (2) File written certifications in the medical record.

[55 FR 50834, Dec. 11, 1990, as amended at 57 FR 36017, Aug. 12, 1992; 70 FR 45144, Aug. 4, 2005; 70 FR 70547, Nov. 22, 2005; 74 FR 39413, Aug. 6, 2009; 75 FR 70463, Nov. 17, 2010; 76 FR 47331, Aug. 4, 2011]

§ 418.24—Election of hospice care.

(a) *Filing an election statement.*

    (1) *General.* An individual who meets the eligibility requirement of § 418.20 may file an election statement with a particular hospice. If the individual is physically or mentally incapacitated, his or her representative (as defined in § 418.3) may file the election statement.

    (2) *Notice of election.* The hospice chosen by the eligible individual (or his or her representative) must file the Notice of Election (NOE) with its Medicare contractor within 5 calendar days after the effective date of the election statement.

    (3) *Consequences of failure to submit a timely notice of election.* When a hospice does not file the required Notice of Election for its Medicare patients within 5 calendar days after the effective date of election, Medicare will not cover and pay for days of hospice care from the effective date of election to the date of filing of the notice of election. These days are a provider liability, and the provider may not bill the beneficiary for them.

    (4) *Exception to the consequences for filing the NOE late.* CMS may waive the consequences of failure to submit a timely-filed NOE specified in paragraph (a)(2) of this section. CMS will determine if a circumstance encountered by a hospice is exceptional and qualifies for waiver of the consequence specified in paragraph (a)(3) of this section. A hospice must fully document and furnish any requested documentation to CMS for a determination of exception. An exceptional circumstance may be due to, but is not limited to the following:

        (i) Fires, floods, earthquakes, or similar unusual events that inflict extensive damage to the hospice's ability to operate.

(ii) A CMS or Medicare contractor systems issue that is beyond the control of the hospice.

(iii) A newly Medicare-certified hospice that is notified of that certification after the Medicare certification date, or which is awaiting its user ID from its Medicare contractor.

(iv) Other situations determined by CMS to be beyond the control of the hospice.

(b) *Content of election statement.* The election statement must include the following:

(1) Identification of the particular hospice and of the attending physician that will provide care to the individual. The individual or representative must acknowledge that the identified attending physician was his or her choice.

(2) The individual's or representative's acknowledgement that he or she has been given a full understanding of the palliative rather than curative nature of hospice care, as it relates to the individual's terminal illness.

(3) Acknowledgement that certain Medicare services, as set forth in paragraph (d) of this section, are waived by the election.

(4) The effective date of the election, which may be the first day of hospice care or a later date, but may be no earlier than the date of the election statement.

(5) The signature of the individual or representative.

(c) *Duration of election.* An election to receive hospice care will be considered to continue through the initial election period and through the subsequent election periods without a break in care as long as the individual

(1) Remains in the care of a hospice;

(2) Does not revoke the election; and

(3) Is not discharged from the hospice under the provisions of § 418.26.

(d) *Waiver of other benefits.* For the duration of an election of hospice care, an individual waives all rights to Medicare payments for the following services:

   (1) Hospice care provided by a hospice other than the hospice designated by the individual (unless provided under arrangements made by the designated hospice).

   (2) Any Medicare services that are related to the treatment of the terminal condition for which hospice care was elected or a related condition or that are equivalent to hospice care except for services

      (i) Provided by the designated hospice;

      (ii) Provided by another hospice under arrangements made by the designated hospice; and

      (iii) Provided by the individual's attending physician if that physician is not an employee of the designated hospice or receiving compensation from the hospice for those services.

(e) *Re-election of hospice benefits.* If an election has been revoked in accordance with § 418.28, the individual (or his or her representative if the individual is mentally or physically incapacitated) may at any time file an election, in accordance with this section, for any other election period that is still available to the individual.

(f) *Changing the attending physician.* To change the designated attending physician, the individual (or representative) must file a signed statement with the hospice that states that he or she is changing his or her attending physician.

   (1) The statement must identify the new attending physician, and include the date the change is to be effective and the date signed by the individual (or representative).

   (2) The individual (or representative) must acknowledge that the change in the attending physician is due to his or her choice.

   (3) The effective date of the change in attending physician cannot be before the date the statement is signed.

[55 FR 50834, Dec. 11, 1990, as amended at 70 FR 70547, Nov. 22, 2005; 79 FR 50509, Aug. 22, 2014]

## § 418.25—Admission to hospice care.

(a) The hospice admits a patient only on the recommendation of the medical director in consultation with, or with input from, the patient's attending physician (if any).

(b) In reaching a decision to certify that the patient is terminally ill, the hospice medical director must consider at least the following information:

    (1) Diagnosis of the terminal condition of the patient.

    (2) Other health conditions, whether related or unrelated to the terminal condition.

    (3) Current clinically relevant information supporting all diagnoses.

[70 FR 70547, Nov. 22, 2005]

## § 418.26—Discharge from hospice care.

(a) *Reasons for discharge.* A hospice may discharge a patient if

    (1) The patient moves out of the hospice's service area or transfers to another hospice;

    (2) The hospice determines that the patient is no longer terminally ill; or

    (3) The hospice determines, under a policy set by the hospice for the purpose of addressing discharge for cause that meets the requirements of paragraphs (a)(3)(i) through (a)(3)(iv) of this section, that the patient's (or other persons in the patient's home) behavior is disruptive, abusive, or uncooperative to the extent that delivery of care to the patient or the ability of the hospice to operate effectively is seriously impaired. The hospice must do the following before it seeks to discharge a patient for cause:

        (i) Advise the patient that a discharge for cause is being considered;

    (ii)  Make a serious effort to resolve the problem(s) presented by the patient's behavior or situation;

    (iii)  Ascertain that the patient's proposed discharge is not due to the patient's use of necessary hospice services; and

    (iv)  Document the problem(s) and efforts made to resolve the problem(s) and enter this documentation into its medical records.

(b) *Discharge order.* Prior to discharging a patient for any reason listed in paragraph (a) of this section, the hospice must obtain a written physician's discharge order from the hospice medical director. If a patient has an attending physician involved in his or her care, this physician should be consulted before discharge and his or her review and decision included in the discharge note.

(c) *Effect of discharge.* An individual, upon discharge from the hospice during a particular election period for reasons other than immediate transfer to another hospice

  (1)  Is no longer covered under Medicare for hospice care;

  (2)  Resumes Medicare coverage of the benefits waived under § 418.24(d); and

  (3)  May at any time elect to receive hospice care if he or she is again eligible to receive the benefit.

(d) *Discharge planning.*

  (1)  The hospice must have in place a discharge planning process that takes into account the prospect that a patient's condition might stabilize or otherwise change such that the patient cannot continue to be certified as terminally ill.

  (2)  The discharge planning process must include planning for any necessary family counseling, patient education, or other services before the patient is discharged because he or she is no longer terminally ill.

(e) *Filing a notice of termination of election.* When the hospice election is ended due to discharge, the hospice must file a notice of termination/revocation of election with its Medicare contractor within 5 calendar days after the effective date of the discharge, unless it has already filed a final claim for that beneficiary.

**[70 FR 70547, Nov. 22, 2005, as amended at 79 FR 50509, Aug. 22, 2014]**

**§ 418.28—Revoking the election of hospice care.**

(a) An individual or representative may revoke the individual's election of hospice care at any time during an election period.

(b) To revoke the election of hospice care, the individual or representative must file a statement with the hospice that includes the following information:

(1) A signed statement that the individual or representative revokes the individual's election for Medicare coverage of hospice care for the remainder of that election period.

(2) The date that the revocation is to be effective. (An individual or representative may not designate an effective date earlier than the date that the revocation is made).

(c) An individual, upon revocation of the election of Medicare coverage of hospice care for a particular election period

(1) Is no longer covered under Medicare for hospice care;

(2) Resumes Medicare coverage of the benefits waived under § 418.24(e)(2); and

(3) May at any time elect to receive hospice coverage for any other hospice election periods that he or she is eligible to receive.

(d) When the hospice election is ended due to revocation, the hospice must file a notice of termination/revocation of election with its Medicare contractor within 5 calendar days after the effective date of the revocation, unless it has already filed a final claim for that beneficiary.

**[48 FR 56026, Dec. 16, 1983, as amended at 79 FR 50509, Aug. 22, 2014]**

**§ 418.30—Change of the designated hospice.**

(a) An individual or representative may change, once in each election period, the designation of the particular hospice from which hospice care will be received.

(b) The change of the designated hospice is not a revocation of the election for the period in which it is made.

(c) To change the designation of hospice programs, the individual or representative must file, with the hospice from which care has been received and with the newly designated hospice, a statement that includes the following information:

  (1) The name of the hospice from which the individual has received care and the name of the hospice from which he or she plans to receive care.

  (2) The date the change is to be effective.

Source: https://www.govregs.com/regulations/expand/title42_chapterIV_part418_subpartB_section418.22#title42_chapterIV_part418_subpartB_section418.20

# Hospice Conditions of Participation: Subpart F— Covered Services

**Title 42 Chapter IV Part 418 - Subpart F - Covered Services**
**§ 418.200—Requirements for coverage.**

To be covered, hospice services must meet the following requirements. They must be reasonable and necessary for the palliation and management of the terminal illness as well as related conditions. The individual must elect hospice care in accordance with § 418.24. A plan of care must be established and periodically reviewed by the attending physician, the medical director, and the interdisciplinary group of the hospice program as set forth in § 418.56. That plan of care must be established before hospice care is provided. The services provided must be consistent with the plan of care. A certification that the individual is terminally ill must be completed as set forth in section § 418.22.

**[74 FR 39413, Aug. 6, 2009]**
**§ 418.202—Covered services.**

All services must be performed by appropriately qualified personnel, but it is the nature of the service, rather than the qualification of the person who provides it, that determines the coverage category of the service. The following services are covered hospice services:

(a) Nursing care provided by or under the supervision of a registered nurse.

(b) Medical social services provided by a social worker under the direction of a physician.

(c) Physicians' services performed by a physician as defined in § 410.20 of this chapter except that the services of the hospice medical director or the physician member of the interdisciplinary group must be performed by a doctor of medicine or osteopathy.

(d) Counseling services provided to the terminally ill individual and the family members or other persons caring for the individual at home. Counseling, including dietary counseling, may be provided both for the purpose of training the individual's family or other caregiver to provide care, and for the purpose of helping the individual and those caring for him or her to adjust to the individual's approaching death.

(e) Short-term inpatient care provided in a participating hospice inpatient unit, or a participating hospital or SNF, that additionally meets the standards in § 418.202 (a) and (e) regarding staffing and patient areas. Services provided in an inpatient setting must conform to the written plan of care. Inpatient care may be required for procedures necessary for pain control or acute or chronic symptom management.

Inpatient care may also be furnished as a means of providing respite for the individual's family or other persons caring for the individual at home. Respite care must be furnished as specified in § 418.108(b). Payment for inpatient care will be made at the rate appropriate to the level of care as specified in § 418.302.

(f) *Medical appliances and supplies, including drugs and biologicals.* Only drugs as defined in section 1861(t) of the Act and which are used primarily for the relief of pain and symptom control related to the individual's terminal illness are covered. Appliances may include covered durable medical equipment as described in § 410.38 of this chapter as well as other self-help and personal comfort items related to the palliation or management of the patient's terminal illness. Equipment is provided by the hospice for use in the patient's home while he or she is under hospice care. Medical supplies include those that are part of the written plan of care and that are for palliation and management of the terminal or related conditions.

(g) *Home health or hospice aide services furnished by qualified aides as designated in § 418.76 and homemaker services.* Home health aides (also known as hospice aides) may provide personal care services as defined in § 409.45(b) of this chapter. Aides may perform household services to maintain a safe and sanitary environment in areas of the home used by the patient, such as changing bed linens or light cleaning and laundering essential to the comfort and cleanliness of the patient. Aide services must be provided under the general supervision of a registered nurse. Homemaker services may include assistance in maintenance of a safe and healthy environment and services to enable the individual to carry out the treatment plan.

(h) Physical therapy, occupational therapy and speech-language pathology services in addition to the services described in § 409.33 (b) and (c) of this chapter provided for purposes of symptom control or to enable the patient to maintain activities of daily living and basic functional skills.

(i) Effective April 1, 1998, any other service that is specified in the patient's plan of care as reasonable and necessary for the palliation and management of the patient's terminal illness and related conditions and for which payment may otherwise be made under Medicare.

[48 FR 56026, Dec. 16, 1983, as amended at 51 FR 41351, Nov. 14, 1986; 55 FR 50835, Dec. 11, 1990; 59 FR 65498, Dec. 20, 1994; 70 FR 70547, Nov. 22, 2005; 73 FR 32220, June 5, 2008; 74 FR 39413, Aug. 6, 2009; 76 FR 47331, Aug. 4, 2011]

### § 418.204—Special coverage requirements.

(a) *Periods of crisis.* Nursing care may be covered on a continuous basis for as much as 24 hours a day during periods of crisis as necessary to maintain an individual at home. Either homemaker or home health aide (also known as hospice aide) services or both may be covered on a 24-hour continuous basis during periods of crisis but care during these periods must be predominantly nursing care. A period of crisis is a period in which the individual requires continuous care to achieve palliation and management of acute medical symptoms.

(b) *Respite care.*

(1) Respite care is short-term inpatient care provided to the individual only when necessary to relieve the family members or other persons caring for the individual.

(2) Respite care may be provided only on an occasional basis and may not be reimbursed for more than five consecutive days at a time.

(c) *Bereavement counseling.* Bereavement counseling is a required hospice service but it is not reimbursable.

[48 FR 56026, Dec. 16, 1983, as amended at 55 FR 50835, Dec. 11, 1990; 74 FR 39413, Aug. 6, 2009]

### § 418.205—Special requirements for hospice pre-election evaluation and counseling services.

(a) *Definition.* As used in this section the following definition applies. *Terminal illness* has the same meaning as defined in § 418.3.

(b) *General.* Effective January 1, 2005, payment for hospice pre-election evaluation and counseling services as specified in § 418.304(d) may be made to a hospice on behalf of a Medicare beneficiary if the requirements of this section are met.

(1) *The beneficiary.* The beneficiary:

   (i) Has been diagnosed as having a terminal illness as defined in § 418.3.

   (ii) Has not made a hospice election.

   (iii) Has not previously received hospice pre-election evaluation and consultation services specified under this section.

(2) *Services provided.* The hospice pre-election services include an evaluation of an individual's need for pain and symptom management and counseling regarding hospice and other care options. In addition, the services may include advising the individual regarding advanced care planning.

(3) *Provision of pre-election hospice services.*

   (i) The services must be furnished by a physician.

   (ii) The physician furnishing these services must be an employee or medical director of the hospice billing for this service.

   (iii) The services cannot be furnished by hospice personnel other than employed physicians, such as but not limited to nurse practitioners, nurses, or social workers, physicians under contractual arrangements with the hospice or by the beneficiary's physician, if that physician is not an employee of the hospice.

   (iv) If the beneficiary's attending physician is also the medical director or a physician employee of the hospice, the attending physician may not provide nor may the hospice bill for this service because that physician already possesses the expertise necessary to furnish end-of-life evaluation and management, and counseling services.

(4) *Documentation.*

   (i) If the individual's physician initiates the request for services of the hospice medical director or physician, appropriate documentation is required.

(ii) The request or referral must be in writing, and the hospice medical director or physician employee is expected to provide a written note on the patient's medical record.

(iii) The hospice agency employing the physician providing these services is required to maintain a written record of the services furnished.

(iv) If the services are initiated by the beneficiary, the hospice agency is required to maintain a record of the services and documentation that communication between the hospice medical director or physician and the beneficiary's physician occurs, with the beneficiary's permission, to the extent necessary to ensure continuity of care.

[69 FR 66425, Nov. 15, 2004]

Source: https://www.govregs.com/regulations/expand/title42_chapterIV_part418_subpartB_section418.22#title42_chapterIV_part418_subpartB_section418.20

# State Hospice and Palliative Care Organizations

**Alabama**
Alabama Hospice & Palliative Care Organization
P.O. Box 26131
Birmingham, AL 35260
(205) 201-2006
www.alhospice.org

**Arizona**
Arizona Hospice & Palliative Care Organization
1850 E. Southern Avenue
Tempe, AZ 85282
(480) 491-0540
www.ahpco.org

**Arkansas**
Hospice & Palliative Care Association of Arkansas
411 S. Victory Street, Suite 205
Little Rock, AR 72201
(501) 375-1300
www.hpcaa.org

### California
California Hospice and Palliative Care Association
3841 N. Freeway Blvd., Suite 100
Sacramento, CA 95834
(916) 925-3770
www.calhospice.org

### Colorado
Hospice & Palliative Care Association of the Rockies
(CO and WY are merged)
2851 S. Parker Road, Suite 1210
Aurora, CO 80014
(303) 848-2522
http://www.hpcar.org/

### Connecticut
Connecticut Association for Healthcare at Home
110 Barnes Road, Box 90
Wallingford, CT 06492
(203) 265-9931
http://www.cthealthcareathome.org/

### Florida
Florida Hospice & Palliative Care Association
2000 Apalachee Parkway, Suite 200
Tallahassee, FL 32301
(850) 878-2632
www.floridahospices.org

### Georgia
Georgia Hospice & Palliative Care Organization
950 Eagles Landing Parkway, Suite 622
Stockbridge, GA 30281
(877) 924-6073
www.ghpco.org

**Hawaii**
Kokua Mau Hawaii Hospice and Palliative Care Organization
P.O. Box 62155
Honolulu, HI 96839
(808) 585-9977
www.kokuamau.org

**Idaho**
Idaho Quality of Life Coalition
P.O. Box 496
Boise, ID 83701
(208) 841-1862
www.idqol.org

**Illinois**
Illinois Hospice & Palliative Care Organization
The PMC Group
902 Ash Street
Winnetka, IL 60093
(847) 441-7200
www.il-hpco.org

Illinois Homecare & Hospice Council
100 E. Washington Street
Springfield, IL 62701
(217) 753-4422
http://www.ilhomecare.org/

**Indiana**
Indiana Hospice & Palliative Care Organization
P.O. Box 68829
Indianapolis, IN 46268-0829
(317) 464-5145
www.ihpco.org

Indiana Association for Home & Hospice Care
6320 Rucker Road, Suite G
Indianapolis, IN 46220
(317) 775-6675
www.iahhc.org

### Iowa
Hospice & Palliative Care Association of Iowa
100 E. Grand Avenue, Suite 120
Des Moines, IA 50309
(515) 243-1046
www.hpcai.org

### Kansas
Kansas Hospice and Palliative Care Organization
313 S. Market Street
Wichita, KS 67220
(316) 207-1764
www.khpco.org

### Kentucky
Kentucky Association of Hospice & Palliative Care
305 Ann Street, Suite 308
Frankfort, KY 40601-2847
(502) 875-1176
www.kah.org

### Louisiana
Louisiana-Mississippi Hospice & Palliative Care Organization
717 Kerlerec Street
New Orleans, LA 70116-2005
(504) 945-2414
www.lmhpco.org

## Maine
Maine Hospice Council & Center for End-of-Life Care
295 Water Street, Suite 303
Augusta, ME 04330
(207) 626-0651
www.mainehospicecouncil.org

## Maryland
Hospice & Palliative Care Network of Maryland
201 International Circle, Suite 230
Hunt Valley, MD 21030
(410) 891-5741
www.hnmd.org

## Massachusetts
Hospice & Palliative Care Federation of Massachusetts
20 Commercial Drive, Suite 1
Wrentham, MA 02093
(781) 255-7077
www.hospicefed.org

## Michigan
Michigan Association for HomeCare & Hospice
2140 University Park Drive, Suite 220
Okemos, MI 48864
Phone: (517) 349-8089  Fax: (517) 349-8090
mhha.org

## Minnesota
Minnesota Network of Hospice & Palliative Care
2365 McKnight Road North, Suite 2
North St. Paul, MN 55109
(651) 917-4616
www.mnhpc.org

**Mississippi**
Louisiana-Mississippi Hospice & Palliative Care Organization
717 Kerlerec Street
New Orleans, LA 70116-2005
(504) 945-2414
www.lmhpco.org

**Missouri**
Missouri Hospice & Palliative Care Association
P.O. Box 105318
Jefferson City, MO 65110
(573) 634-5514
www.mohospice.org

**Montana**
MHA an Association of Montana Healthcare Providers
2625 Winne Avenue
Helena, MT 59601
(406) 442-1911
www.mtha.org

**Nebraska**
Nebraska Hospice & Palliative Care Association
1200 Libra Drive, Suite 100
Lincoln, NE 68512
(402) 477-0204
www.nehospice.org

**New Hampshire**
New Hampshire Hospice and Palliative Care Organization
125 Airport Road
Concord, NH 03301
(603) 415-4298
www.nhhpco.org

**New Jersey**
New Jersey Hospice and Palliative Care Organization
1044 Route 22 West, Suite 2
Mountainside, NJ 07092
(908) 233-0060
www.njhospice.org

**New Mexico**
Texas & New Mexico Hospice Organization
1108 Lavaca, Suite 727
Austin, TX 78701
(512) 454-1247
www.txnmhospice.org

**New York**
Hospice & Palliative Care Association of New York State
2 Computer Drive West, Suite 105
Albany, NY 12205
(518) 446-1483
http://www.hpcanys.org/

**North Carolina**
Carolinas Center for Hospice & End of Life Care
8502 Six Forks Road, Suite 101
Raleigh, NC 27615
(919) 459-5380
www.cchospice.org

Association for Home & Hospice Care of North Carolina
3101 Industrial Drive, Suite 204
Raleigh, NC 27609
(919) 848-3450
www.homeandhospicecare.org

## Ohio

LeadingAge Ohio
2233 N. Bank Drive
Columbus, OH 43220
(614) 444-2882
www.midwestcarealliance.org

## Oklahoma

Oklahoma Hospice & Palliative Care Association
P.O. Box 1466
Ardmore, OK 73402
(405) 513-8602
http://www.okhospice.org/

## Oregon

Oregon Hospice & Palliative Care Association
P.O. Box 592
Marylhurst, OR 97036
(503) 228-2104
www.oregonhospice.org

## Pennsylvania

Pennsylvania Hospice and Palliative Care Network
475 W. Governor Road, Suite 7
Hershey, PA 17033
(717) 533-4002
www.pahospice.org

Pennsylvania Homecare Association
600 N. 12th Street, Suite 200
Lemoyne, PA 17043
(800) 382-1211
www.pahomecare.org

**South Carolina**
Carolinas Center for Hospice & End of Life Care
1350 Browning Road
Columbia, SC 29210
(803) 509-1021
http://cchospice.org/

South Carolina Home Care & Hospice Association
3101 Industrial Drive, Suite 204
Raleigh, NC 27609
(919) 848-3450
www.schomehealth.org

**Tennessee**
Tennessee Hospice Organization
5201 Virginia Way
Brentwood, TN 37027
(615) 401-7469
www.tnhospice.org

**Texas**
Texas & New Mexico Hospice Organization
1108 Lavaca, Suite 727
Austin, TX 78701
(512) 454-1247
www.txnmhospice.org

**Utah**
Utah Hospice & Palliative Care Organization
1327 S. 900 East
Salt Lake City, UT 84105-2301
(801) 582-2245
http://utahhospice.org/

**Vermont**
Hospice and Palliative Care Council of Vermont
137 Elm Street #3
Montpelier, VT 05602
(802) 229-0579
http://www.hpccv.org/

**Virginia**
Virginia Association for Hospices & Palliative Care
P.O. Box 70025
Richmond, VA 23255
(804) 740-1344
www.virginiahospices.org

**Washington**
Washington State Hospice & Palliative Care Organization
P.O. Box 361
Camas, WA 98607
(253) 661-3739
https://wshpco.org/

**West Virginia**
Hospice Council of West Virginia
1804 Rolling Hills Road
Charleston, WV 25314
(304) 206-8929
www.hospicecouncilofwv.org

**Wisconsin**
The HOPE of Wisconsin
3240 University Avenue, Suite 2
Madison, WI 53705-3570
(608) 233-7166
https://www.hopeofwisconsin.org/

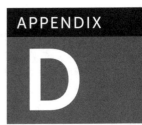

# Resources

## Centers for Medicare and Medicaid Services (CMS)

CMS Local Coverage Determinations (LCDs) by State (https://www.cms.gov/medicare-coverage-database/indexes/lcd-state-index.aspx?s=All&DocType=Active%7CFuture&Cntrctr=247&ContrVer=1&CntrctrSelected=247*1&name=Noridian+Administrative+Services%2C+LLC+(02402%2C+MAC+-+Part+B)&bc=AggAAAAAAAAAA%3D%3D&#ResultsAnchor)

Hospice Center (https://www.cms.gov/Center/Provider-Type/Hospice-Center.html)

Medicare Benefit Policy Manual Chapter 9: Coverage of Hospice Services Under Hospital Insurance (https://www.cms.gov/Regulations-and-Guidance/Guidance/Manuals/Downloads/bp102c09.pdf)

Medicare Claims Processing Manual Chapter 11: Processing Hospice Claims (https://www.cms.gov/Regulations-and-Guidance/Guidance/Manuals/Downloads/clm104c11.pdf)

State Operations Manual Chapter 2: The Certification Process (https://www.cms.gov/Regulations-and-Guidance/Guidance/Manuals/downloads/som107c02.pdf)

## Trade Organizations

American Academy of Hospice and Palliative Medicine (http://aahpm.org)

Center to Advance Palliative Care (CAPC) (capc.org)

National Association for Home Care & Hospice (NAHC) (http://www.nahc.org/) (202) 547-7424

National Hospice and Palliative Care Organization (NHPCO) (www.nhpco.org) (703) 837-1500

Visiting Nurse Associations of America (VNAA) (www.vnaa.org) (571) 527-1520

World Health Organization (http://www.who.int/en/)

## Other Resources

Aging with Dignity
http://www.agingwithdignity.org/five-wishes.php

Eastern Cooperative Oncology Group Performance Status
ecog-acrin.org/resources/ecog-performance-status

Flacker Mortality Score
http://www.ucdenver.edu/academics/colleges/medicalschool/departments/medicine/hcpr/palliativecare/mortalitytools/Documents/Flacker%20Mortality%20Score.pdf

Hospice Eligibility Information Card with Palliative Performance Scale
http://geriatrics.uthscsa.edu/tools/Hospice_elegibility_card__Ross_and_Sanchez_Reilly_2008.pdf

JAMA Evidence: Care at the Close of Life
http://www.jamaevidence.com/resource/648

Karnofsky Performance Scale
http://endoflife.stanford.edu/media/karnofsky.htm

Palliative Care Information Resources
http://palliative.info/pages/education.htm

Palliative Prognostic Score
https://www.mypcnow.org/blank-h1jat

Physician Orders for Life-Sustaining Treatment Paradigm
www.polst.org

# Index

# W

# Y